ANATOMY
TO COLOR
AND STUDY
HEAD
AND
NECK
3rd edition

Ray Poritsky, Ph.D. Emeritus
Department of Anatomy
Case Western University School of Medicine
Cleveland, Ohio

ISBN: 978-0-9835784-4-4
Copyright © 2011 Ray Poritsky
Digitally Reproduced by:
CONVERPAGE
23 Acorn Street
Scituate, MA 02066
www.converpage.com

All rights reserved. No part of this publication may be reproduced, stored in a retrieval system, or transmitted, in any form or by any means, electronic, mechanical, photocopying, recording or otherwise, without the written prior permission of the author.

CONTENTS

Head and Neck

1. Superficial muscles of the face and neck
2. Muscles of facial expression
3. Superficial structures on the lateral head
4. Bones of the skull, anterior aspect
5. Bones of the skull, lateral aspect
6. Facial nerve
7. Landmarks on the lateral skull
8. Temporalis and masseter muscles
9. Temporalis muscle
10. Buccinator and orbicularis oris muscles
11. Median section of skull and mandible
12. Interior of the skull
13. Superficial veins of the head and neck
14. External carotid artery and its branches

Cartoon: Sagitta

15. Cranial dural venous sinuses
16. Head and neck: midsagittal aspect
17. Superior sagittal sinus
18. Interior of the skull with cranial nerve exits
19. Facial nerve and its branches
20. Functional components of the facial nerve
21. Inferior surface of skull

Cartoon: Temporal

22. Sphenoid bone
23. Temporal bone, external surface
24. Temporal bone, internal surface
25. Superficial muscles of the neck
26. Left side of neck I
27. Left side of neck II
28. Mandibular nerve and maxillary artery I
29. Mandibular nerve and maxillary artery II
30. The eyelid and eye in orbit
31. Extraocular muscles
32. Eye and orbit
33. Nerves of the orbit, superior aspect
34. Nerves of the orbit, lateral aspect
35. Lower half of right eye
36. Principal veins of face and orbit
37. The lacrimal apparatus
38. Dissection of ear and cast of bony labyrinth
39. Dissection of ear
40. Middle ear and ear ossicles
41. Ear ossicles and part of eardrum
42. Middle ear ossicles
43. Dissection of right ear showing middle ear and cochlea
44. Membranous labyrinth of left inner ear cut open
45. Dissection of right temporal bone showing sigmoid sinus and facial canal
46. Section through external ear, middle ear, and inner ear

Cartoon: Tragus

47. Cartilages of the nose
48. Nasal cavity, lateral wall
49. Nasal cavity, bones and cartilages
50. Nasal cavity, lateral wall and frontal section
51. Pterygopalatine ganglion
52. Olfactory nerves and arterial supply of nasal cavity
53. Right wall of nasal cavity and ethmoidal air cells
54. Projection of paranasal sinuses on front and side of face
55. Oral and nasal cavities in sagittal section
56. Skull, coronal section
57. Sagittal section of head
58. Pharynx
59. Muscles of the tongue, pharynx, and larynx
60. Oral cavity
61. Tongue I
62. Tongue II
63. Tongue and related structures, coronal section
64. Temporomandibular joint

Cartoon: Latin words used to describe parts of the nervous system

65. Mandible
66. Salivary glands
67. Oral cavity, from inside
68. Infratemporal fossa
69. Maxillary artery
70. Muscles of the pharynx
71. Arytenoid and cricoid cartilages
72. Vocal ligaments and muscles
73. Larynx, cartilages
74. Pharynx, posterior aspect
75. Arytenoid cartilages
76. Larynx, cartilages, posterior aspect
77. Larynx, nerves and muscles
78. Larynx, coronal section
79. Muscle origins and insertions on side of skull
80. Skull, inferior aspect
81. Autonomic outflow in the head I
82. Autonomic outflow in the head II

Cartoon: Synapse

83. Inferior view of the brain
84. Medial view of right half of brain
85. The cranial nerves
86. Brain stem
87. Arterial supply at base of brain

Cartoon: Thalamus means bedroom

88. Head frontal section: level of eyes and nasal cavity
89. Head frontal section: level of eye muscles, sinuses
90. Head frontal section: level of maxillary sinuses
91. Head frontal section: level of sphenoid sinuses
92. Head frontal section: level of optic chiasm level
93. Head frontal section: level of carotid canal
94. Head frontal section: level of pons, internal jugular vein
95. Head frontal section: level of dens of axis
96. Cartoon: Trigemini (triplets)

This book allows the reader to learn human anatomy in a simple and direct manner by coloring and labeling key anatomical structures. Many students will be engaged in anatomical dissection in the gross anatomy laboratory (the word *anatomy* comes from the Greek "to cut").

These plates cover the seven regions of the body. The traditional color scheme of anatomy textbooks and atlases is red for arteries, blue for veins, yellow for nerves, pink to reddish brown for muscles, and white or light tan for bones. The reader will find that good quality sharp color pencils work quite well.

There is very little explanatory text. In a few places, short paragraphs have been added that impart important aspects of applied anatomy. Etymological cartoons are interspersed throughout for a brief change and convey some information about Latin and Greek roots.

Color pencils ready... go!

Ray Poritsky, Ph.D.

ACKNOWLEDGMENTS

Many of the illustrations were drawn by the author, who has had formal training in anatomy and medical illustration. Additional drawings were done by Helen Williams, Susan Weil, Cheryl Owens, and James Bille. The author used the following texts as source materials: Spalteholz and Spanner: *Atlas of Human Anatomy, 16th ed.*, Philadelphia, F.A. Davis, 1961; Wolf-Heidegger: *Atlas of Systematic Human Anatomy*, New York, Hafner, 1962; Hollinshead and Rosse: *Textbook of Anatomy, 4th ed.*, Philadelphia, Harper and Row, 1985; Netter: *The Ciba Collection of Medical Illustrations*, Summit, NJ, Ciba Pharmaceutical Company, 1959, 1962; Clemente: *Anatomy: A Regional Atlas of the Human Body, 3rd ed.*, Baltimore and Munich, Urban & Schwarzenberg, 1987; Rohen and Yokochi: *Color Atlas of Anatomy: A Photographic Study of the Human Body*, New York and Tokyo, Igaku-Shoin, 1984; Moore: *Clinically Oriented Anatomy*, Baltimore, Williams & Wilkins, 1982; Clemente: *Anatomy of the Human Body, 13th ed.*, Philadelphia, Lea & Febiger, 1985; Williams and Warwick: *Gray's Anatomy, 36th British ed.*, Edinburgh, Churchill Livingstone, 1980; Anson: *Morris' Human Anatomy: A Complete Systematic Treatise, 12th ed.*, New York, McGraw-Hill, 1966; Pernkopf: *Atlas of Topographical and Applied Human Anatomy*, Munich, Urban & Schwarzenberg, 1980. I also found certain Somso anatomical models most helpful for several of the drawings.

The following sources were employed for the section on The Upper Limb and The Lower Limb and are gratefully acknowledged. Several figures were drawn by Cheryl Owens and Wayne Timmerman. Illustrations are reworked and updated figures from Eycleshymer and Jones: *Hand Atlas of Clinical Anatomy*, Lea & Febiger, 1925. Other atlases and texts consulted include: Wolf-Heidegger: *Atlas of Systemic Human Anatomy*, Hafner, 1962; Spalteholz and Spanner: *Atlas of Human Anatomy, 16th ed.*, F.A. Davis, 1961; Hollinshead and Rosse: *Textbook of Anatomy, 4th ed.*, Harper and Row, 1985; Clemente: *A Regional Atlas of the Human Body, 3rd ed.*, Urban & Schwarzenberg, 1987; Töndury: *Angewandte und Topographische Anatomie*, Fretz & Wasmuth, 1949; Williams (ed): *Gray's Anatomy, 38th British ed.*, Churchill Livingstone, 1995; Netter: *The Ciba Collection of Medical Illustrations*, Ciba Pharmaceutical Company, 1959.

I thank and warmly dedicate this book to my wife Connie.

H&N-1 Superficial muscles of the face and neck

1 _____
2 _____
3 _____
4 _____
5 _____
6 _____
7 _____
8 _____
9 _____
10 _____
11 _____
12 _____
13 _____
14 _____
15 _____
16 _____
17 _____
18 _____
19 _____
20 _____

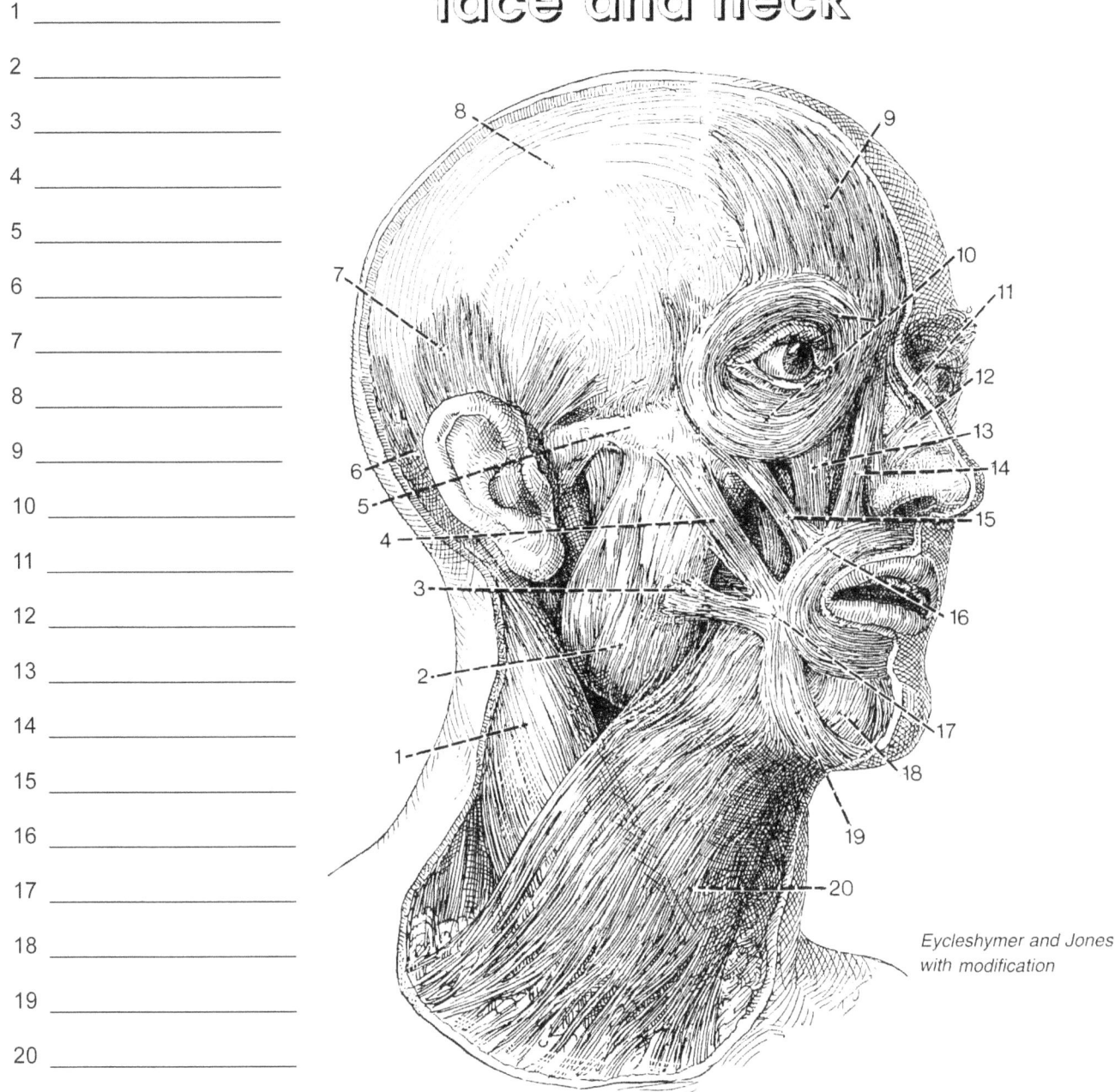

Eycleshymer and Jones with modification

Color and label

1. Sternocleidomastoid
2. Masseter
3. Risorius
4. Zygomaticus major
5. Zygomatic arch (also, zygoma)
6. Occipitalis
7. Superior auricular
8. Galea aponeurotica (also, epicranial aponeurosis)
9. Frontalis (also, frontal belly of occipitofrontalis)
10. Orbicularis oculi (orbital part)
11. Procerus
12. Nasalis (transverse part)
13. Levator labii superioris (also, levator muscle of upper lip)
14. Levator labii superioris alaeque nasi (also, levator muscle of upper lip and ala of nose)
15. Zygomaticus minor
16. Orbicularis oris (marginal part)
17. Modiolus
18. Depressor labii inferioris (also, depressor of lower lip)
19. Depressor anguli oris (also, depressor of angle of mouth)
20. Platysma

H&N-2 Muscles of facial expression
(opposite page)

Color and label

1. Galea aponeurotica (*galea*, L. a helmet); the tough, fibrous cap-like membrane covering the top of the skull anchored on each side by 3 paired muscles that make up the epicranial muscle: the occipitalis, the frontalis, and the temporoparietalis (also called epicranial aponeurosis; cut edge indicated at *).
2. Frontal belly of occipitofrontalis muscle
3. Temporoparietalis muscle (highly variable)
4. Orbicularis oculi muscle (also called orbicular muscle of the eye, sphincter of eye)
    - 4A Orbital part (cut on left side of face)
    - 4B Palpebral part (cut on left side)
    - 4C Origin of medial orbital part

    The upper and lower eyelids are each a fold of reinforced skin that consists of (from without inward): skin, areolar tissue, orbicularis oculi muscle, tarsus, orbital septum, tarsal glands, and conjunctiva (a membrane that lines both the inside of the eyelid and the outer surface of the eyeball; the upper and lower eyelids close the eye and wink the eye.
5. Medial palpebral ligament
6. Superior tarsus of eyelid (a plate of condensed fibrous tissue); its orbital margin is attached to the superior orbit by the orbital septum.
7. Inferior tarsus of eyelid (a plate of condensed fibrous tissue); its orbital margin is attached to the lower orbit by the orbital septum.
8. Orbital septum; a thin, fibrous sheath lining the inner surface of the orbicularis oculi muscle and blending with the aponeurosis of the levator palpebrae superioris muscle in the upper eyelid.
9. Tendon of levator palpebrae superioris muscle
10. Corrugator supercilli; produces a vertical furrow, the frowning muscle.
11. Procerus muscle; it pulls down the medial end of the eyebrows, producing transverse wrinkles above the root of the nose.
12. Auricularis anterior; in humans the three auricular muscles of the external ear are rather weak movers of the ears, unlike the auricular muscles in most mammals.
13. Zygomaticus major; pulls the angle of the mouth upward and laterally.
14. Zygomaticus minor; raises the outer part of the upper lip and accentuates the nasolabial fold.
15. Levator labii superioris; raises and everts the upper lip.
16. Levator labii superioris alaeque nasi; its medial part dilates the nostril, and its lateral part raises and everts the upper lip, and elevates the nasolabial fold.
17. Levator anguli oris; raises the angle of the mouth.
18. Masseter; a muscle of mastication; a strong closer of the jaw, innervated by the trigeminal nerve (cranial nerve V)
19. Parotid duct
20. Risorius; pulls the angle of the mouth laterally.
21. Nasalis
    - 21A Transverse part; compresses the nasal septum.
    - 21B Alar part; this part pulls the wings (alae) of the nose downwards and laterally, dilating the nostrils.
22. Depressor septi
23. Orbicularis oris (also called the orbicular muscle of the mouth); it closes the mouth, compresses the lips against the teeth, and protrudes the lips.
    - 23A Marginal part; this part blends with eight surrounding muscles that converge and interlace at the modiolus at each angle of the mouth.
    - 23B Labial part; this part lies within the lips.
24. Depressor anguli oris
25. Depressor labii inferior
26. Mentalis; draws up and wrinkles the skin of the chin, protruding the lower lip.
27. Buccinator; flattens the cheeks, and pulls the angle of the mouth laterally (*buccinator* means trumpeter in Latin)
28. Platysma; a thin broad muscle covering most of the anterior neck; pulls the lower lip and mouth laterally and inferiorly, partially opening the mouth
29. Outline of masseter

The facial muscles of expression (or muscles of facial expression) are unusual in that they insert not on bone, but on the skin of the face. By pulling on the skin, especially that around the eyes and mouth, they are able to express one's feelings and emotions. They are all innervated by the facial nerve, even the platysma which is largely in the neck. At their insertions they tend to blend and intertwine with neighboring facial muscles.

H&N-2 Muscles of facial expression

1 _____
2 _____
3 _____
4 _____
5 _____
6 _____
7 _____
8 _____
9 _____
10 _____
11 _____
12 _____
13 _____
14 _____
15 _____
16 _____
17 _____
18 _____
19 _____
20 _____
21 _____
22 _____
23 _____
24 _____
25 _____
26 _____
27 _____
28 _____
29 _____

(Use abbrevs.)

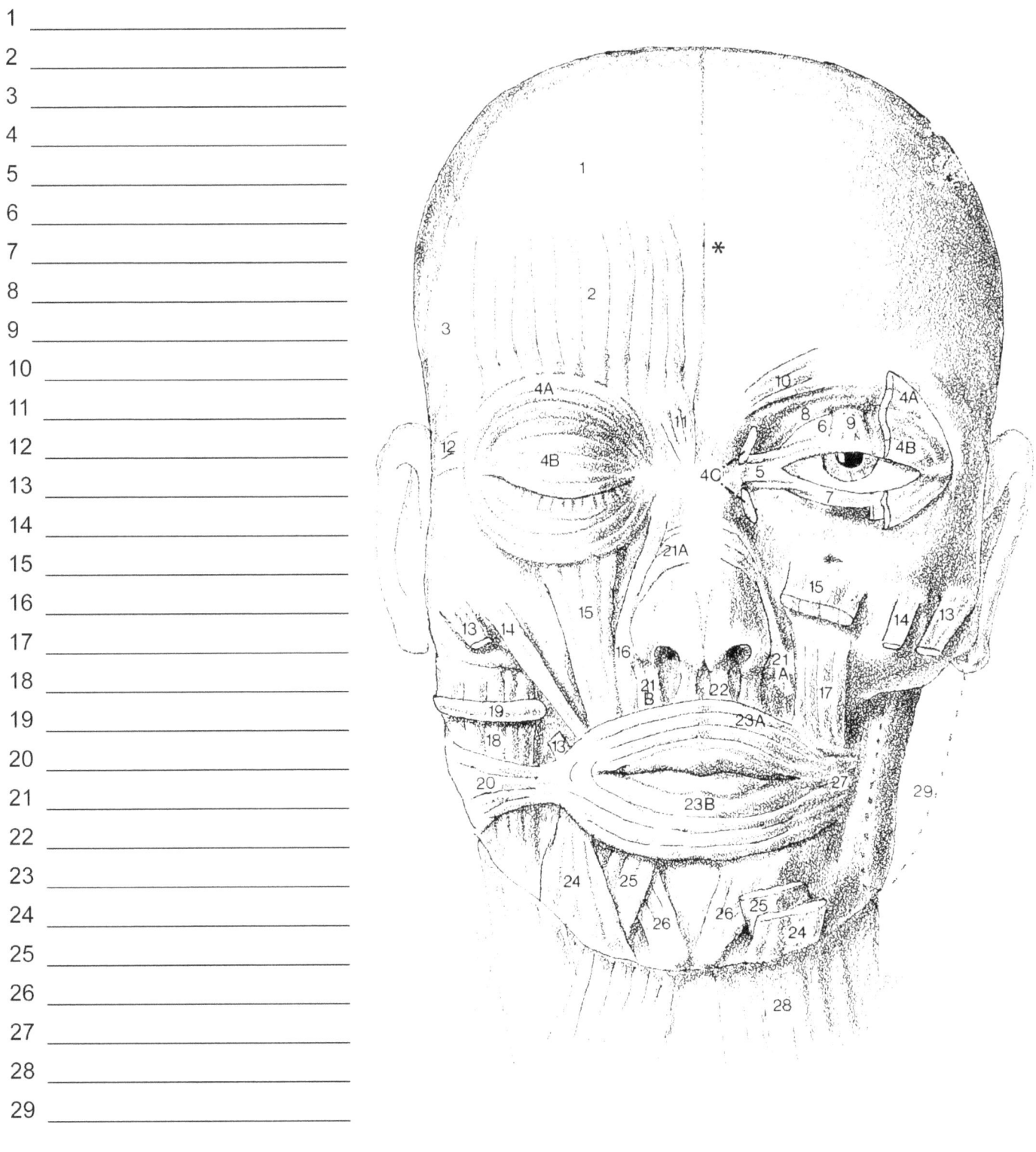

H&N-3 Superficial structures of the lateral head

(opposite page)

Color and label

1. Parotid gland
2. Parotid duct
3. Temporal branches of the facial nerve
4. Zygomatic branches of facial nerve
5. Buccal branches of facial nerve
6. Marginal mandibular branch of facial nerve
7. Cervical branch of facial nerve
8. Transverse facial artery
9. Facial artery and vein
10. Superficial temporal artery and vein
11. Auriculotemporal nerve; a branch of the mandibular nerve (of nerve V)
12. External jugular vein
13. Great auricular nerve
14. Transverse cervical nerves
15. Supraclavicular nerve
16. Lesser occipital nerve
17. Accessory parotid gland
18. Buccal fat pad
19. Accessory nerve (cranial nerve XI)
20. Angular artery and vein
21. Masseter muscle
22. Orbicularis oculi muscle
23. Zygomaticus major muscle
24. Zygomaticus minor muscle
25. Platysma muscle
26. Sternocleidomastoid muscle
27. Trapezius muscle
28. Occipital artery
29. Greater occipital nerve
30. Modiolus (or modiolus labii); a nodular mass of decussating muscles mainly from the upper and lower lips interlacing with other facial muscles such as the buccinator (which has been removed).

1 _____
2 _____
3 _____
4 _____
5 _____
6 _____
7 _____
8 _____
9 _____
10 _____

11 _____
12 _____
13 _____
14 _____
15 _____
16 _____
17 _____
18 _____
19 _____
20 _____
21 _____
22 _____
23 _____
24 _____
25 _____
26 _____
27 _____
28 _____
29 _____
30 _____

H&N-3 Superficial structures of the lateral head

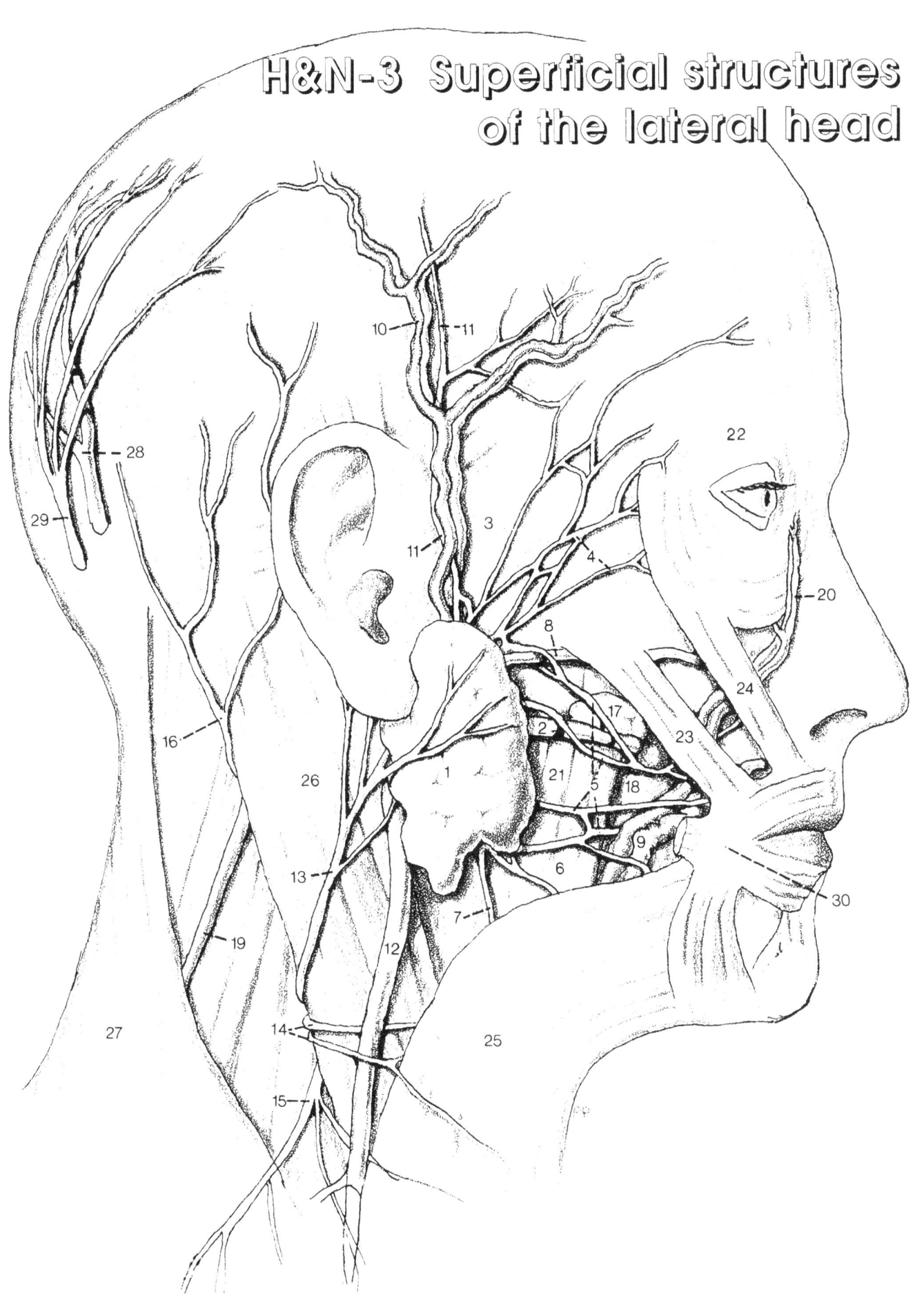

H&N-4 Bones of the skull
Anterior aspect

Color and label these bones

1. Frontal bone
   - 1A Squamous part
   - 1B Orbital part
2. Sphenoid bone
   - 2A Greater wing, orbital surface
   - 2B Lesser wing
   - 2C Greater wing, temporal surface
3. Zygomatic bone
   - 3A Lateral surface
   - 3B Frontal process
   - 3C Orbital surface
4. Maxillary bone (maxilla)
   - 4A Body
   - 4B Nasal process
   - 4C Orbital surface
5. Mandible
   - 5A Mental protuberance
   - 5B Body
   - 5C Ramus
6. Nasal bone
7. Temporal bone
   - 7A Squamous part
   - 7B Mastoid process
   - 7C Zygomatic process
8. Inferior nasal concha
9. Lacrimal bone
10. Parietal bone
11. Vomer
12. Ethoid bone
    - 12A Perpendicular plate
    - 12B Middle nasal concha

Label these foramina

13. Optic canal
14. Superior orbital fissure
15. Inferior orbital fissure
16. Infraorbital groove
17. Supraorbital foramen (sometimes just a notch)
18. Infraorbital foramen
19. Mental foramen

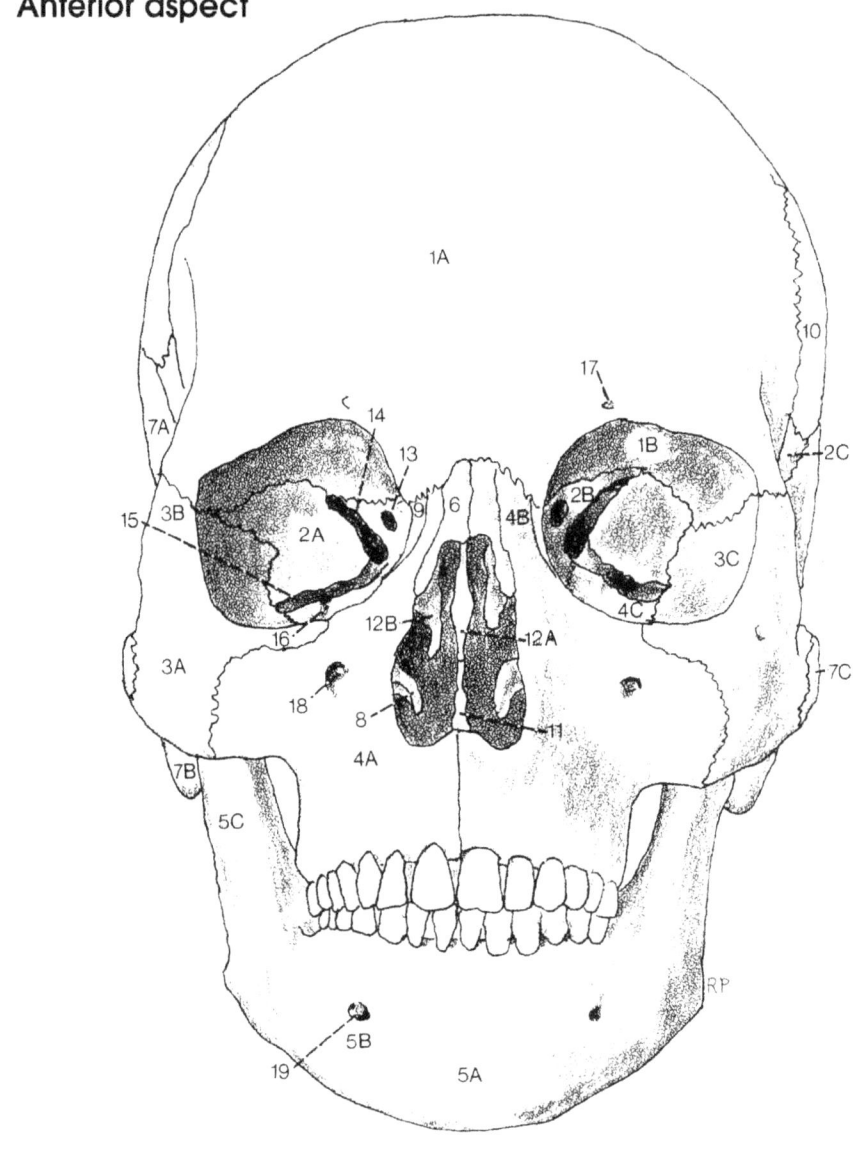

1 _____
2 _____
3 _____
4 _____
5 _____
6 _____
7 _____
8 _____
9 _____
10 _____
11 _____
12 _____
13 _____
14 _____
15 _____
16 _____
17 _____
18 _____
19 _____

H&N-5 Bones of the skull

Lateral aspect

Color and label

1 Mental protuberance
2 Mental foramen
3 Infraorbital foramen
4 Neck of mandible (head of mandible forms temporomandibular joint with temporal bone)
5 Coronoid process
6 Mastoid process of temporal bone
7 External auditory meatus
8 Lambdoidal suture
9 Squamous suture
10 Coronal suture

S Sphenoid bone
F Frontal bone
L Lacrimal bone
N Nasal bone
Max Maxillary bone
P Parietal bone
O Occipital bone
T Temporal bone
Z Zygomatic bone
E Ethmoid bone
M Mandible

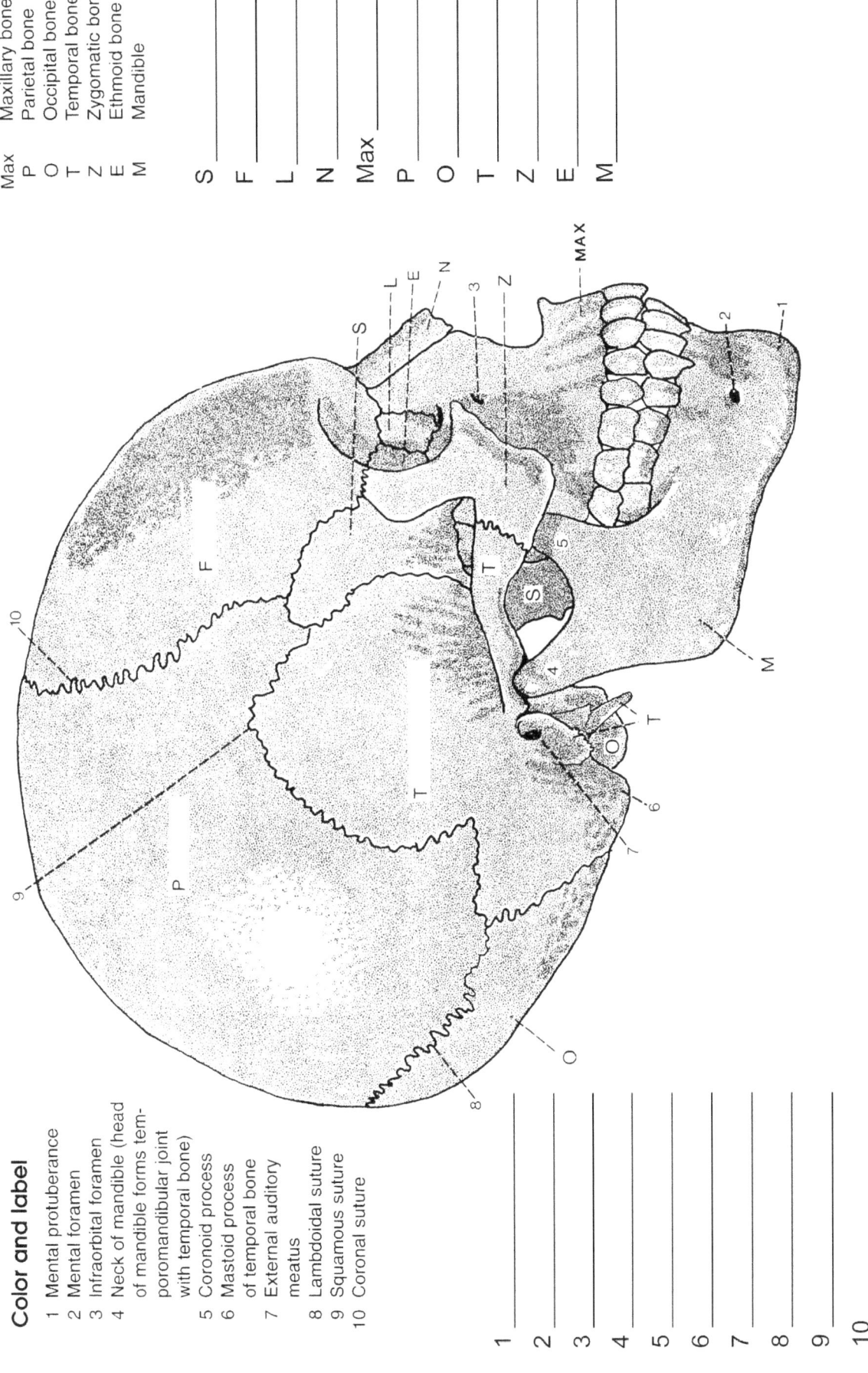

S ____
F ____
L ____
N ____
Max ____
P ____
O ____
T ____
Z ____
E ____
M ____

1 ____
2 ____
3 ____
4 ____
5 ____
6 ____
7 ____
8 ____
9 ____
10 ____

H&N-6 Facial nerve

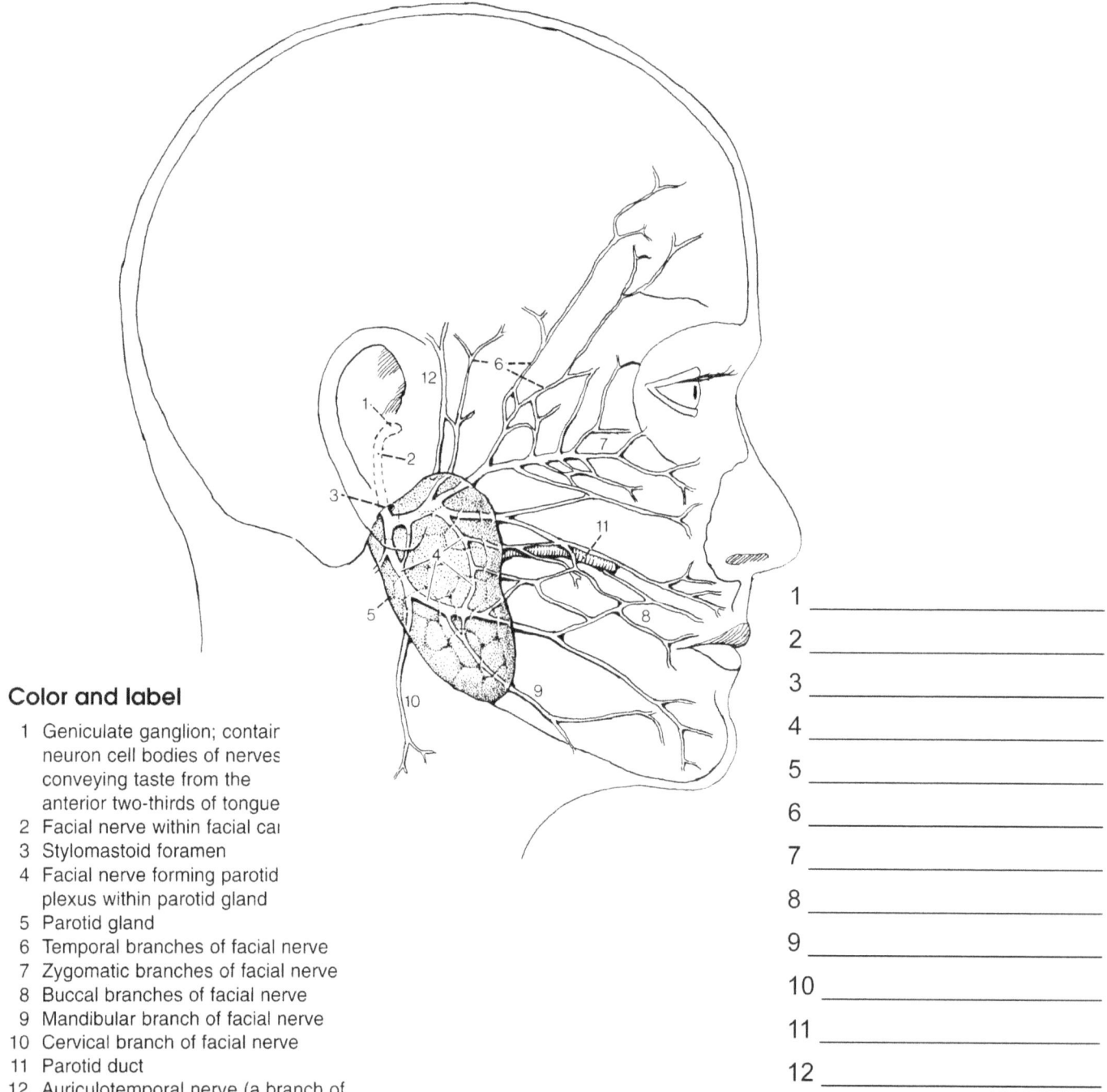

Color and label

1. Geniculate ganglion; contains neuron cell bodies of nerves conveying taste from the anterior two-thirds of tongue
2. Facial nerve within facial canal
3. Stylomastoid foramen
4. Facial nerve forming parotid plexus within parotid gland
5. Parotid gland
6. Temporal branches of facial nerve
7. Zygomatic branches of facial nerve
8. Buccal branches of facial nerve
9. Mandibular branch of facial nerve
10. Cervical branch of facial nerve
11. Parotid duct
12. Auriculotemporal nerve (a branch of the mandibular nerve)

SUPERFICIAL MOTOR BRANCHES

*The parotid plexus has been given the name *pes anserinus*, or goose's foot, for its supposed resemblance to the webbed foot of a goose.

The facial nerve consists of a **motor root** and a distinct **nervus intermedius**. The latter carries sensory fibers (largely taste) and parasympathetic preganglionic fibers. The facial nerve supplies the muscles of facial expression, the muscles of the scalp and auricle, the buccinator, the platysma, the posterior belly of the digastric, the stylohyoid, and the tiny stapedius muscle in the middle ear. After leaving the brain stem, the facial nerve passes through the rather long bony facial canal within the temporal bone. Emerging from the canal at the stylomastoid foramen, it then enters the parotid gland in which it ramifies, its branches forming a plexus, the parotid plexus,* which gives off branches to the facial expression muscles. The facial nerve's motor branches from the parotid plexus to the facial muscles travel close to the skin. Damage to the facial nerve results in Bell's palsy (unilateral paralysis of facial muscles supplied by the seventh nerve).

H&N-7 Landmarks on the lateral skull

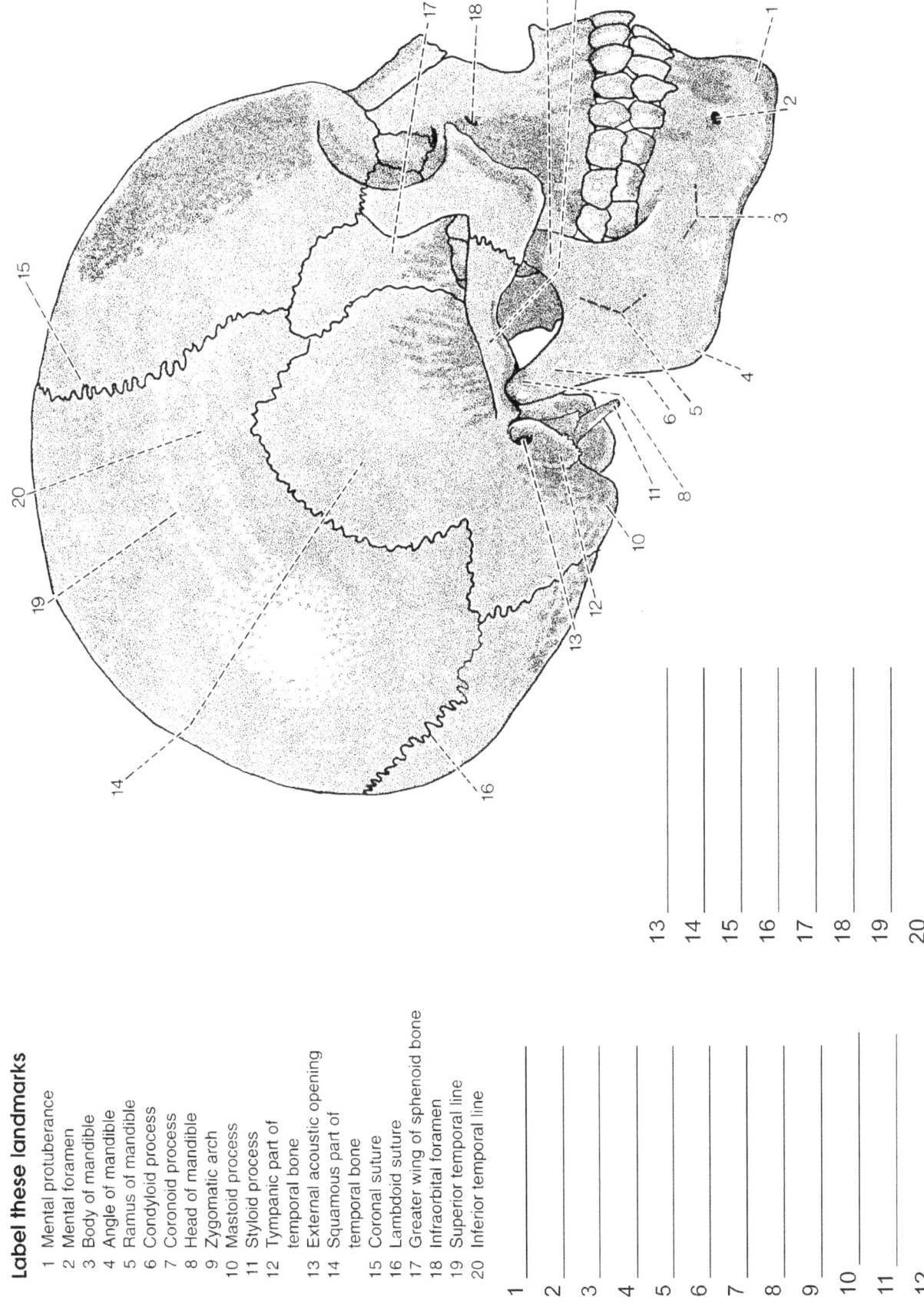

Label these landmarks

1. Mental protuberance
2. Mental foramen
3. Body of mandible
4. Angle of mandible
5. Ramus of mandible
6. Condyloid process
7. Coronoid process
8. Head of mandible
9. Zygomatic arch
10. Mastoid process
11. Styloid process
12. Tympanic part of temporal bone
13. External acoustic opening
14. Squamous part of temporal bone
15. Coronal suture
16. Lambdoid suture
17. Greater wing of sphenoid bone
18. Infraorbital foramen
19. Superior temporal line
20. Inferior temporal line

1 _____
2 _____
3 _____
4 _____
5 _____
6 _____
7 _____
8 _____
9 _____
10 _____
11 _____
12 _____
13 _____
14 _____
15 _____
16 _____
17 _____
18 _____
19 _____
20 _____

H&N-8 Temporalis and masseter muscles

Color and label

1 Temporalis muscle
2 Masseter muscle
3 Deep part of masseter

The temporalis, masseter, medial and lateral pterygoids are the muscles of mastication (chewing). They are innervated by nerve V, the trigeminal nerve.

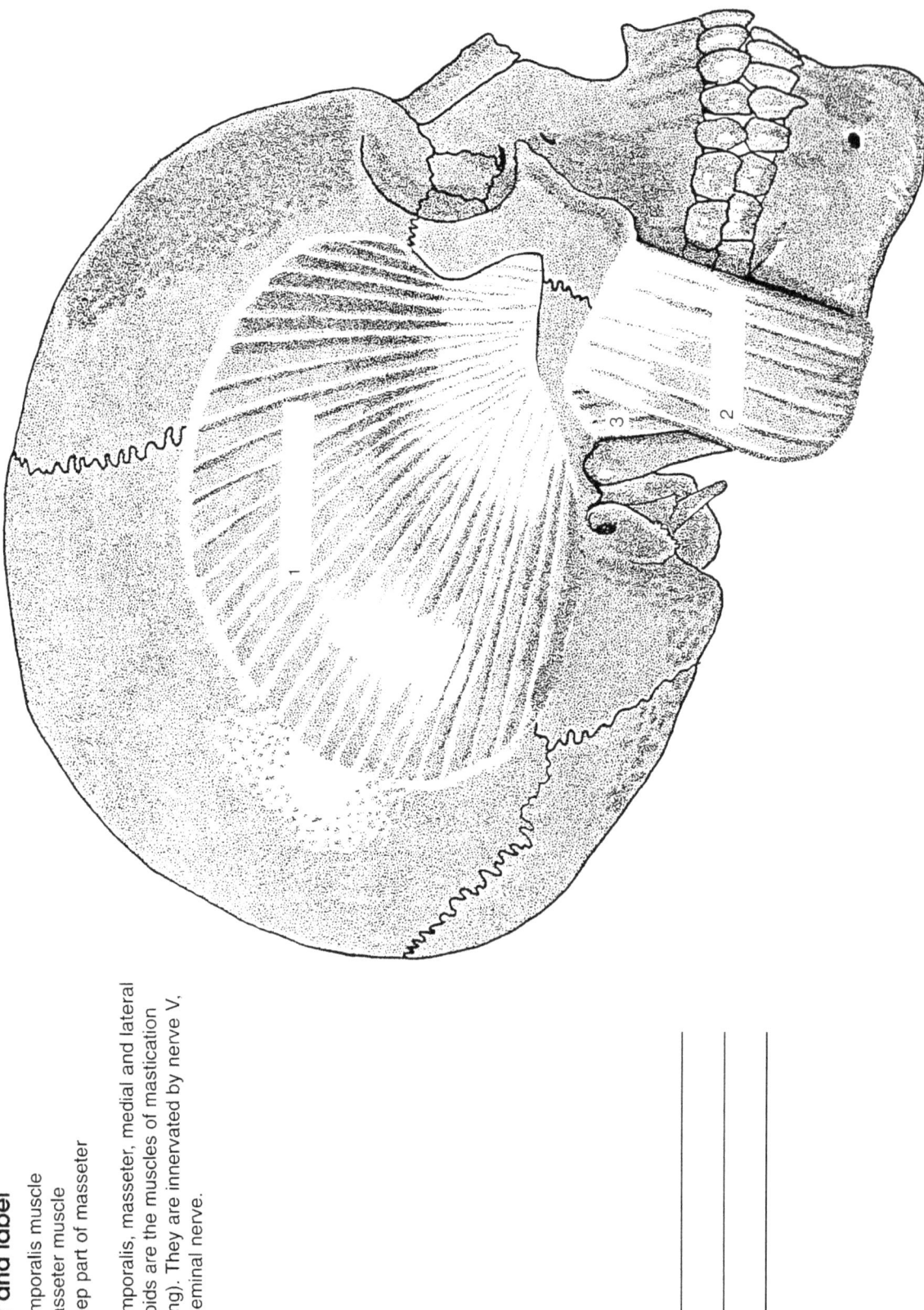

1 _____
2 _____
3 _____

H&N-9 Temporalis muscle

Color and label

1. Temporalis muscle
2. Insertion of temporalis on coronoid process and ramus of mandible
3. Zygomatic arch (cut)
4. Insertion of masseter on ramus and angle of mandible

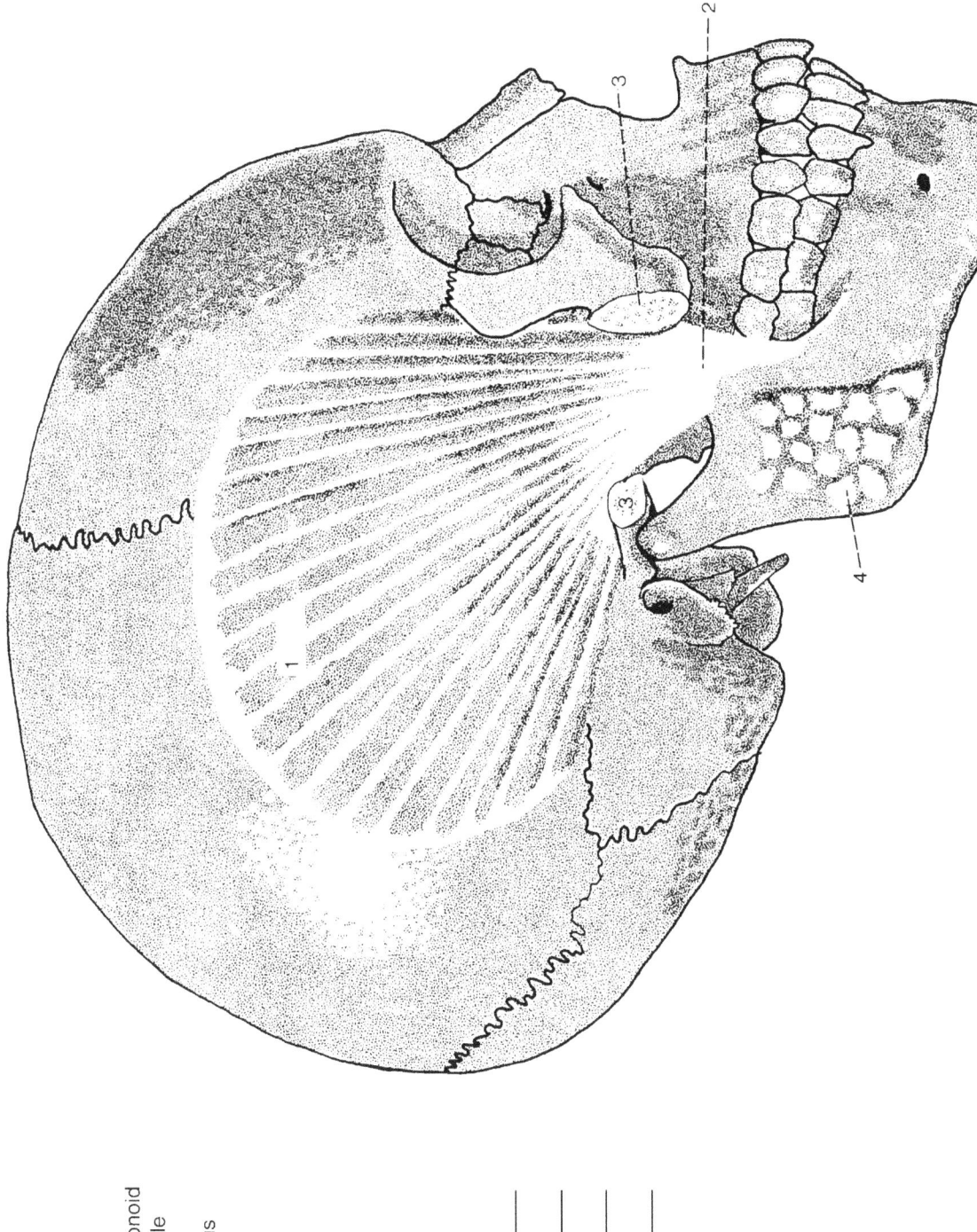

1 _____
2 _____
3 _____
4 _____

H&N-10 Buccinator and orbicularis oris muscles

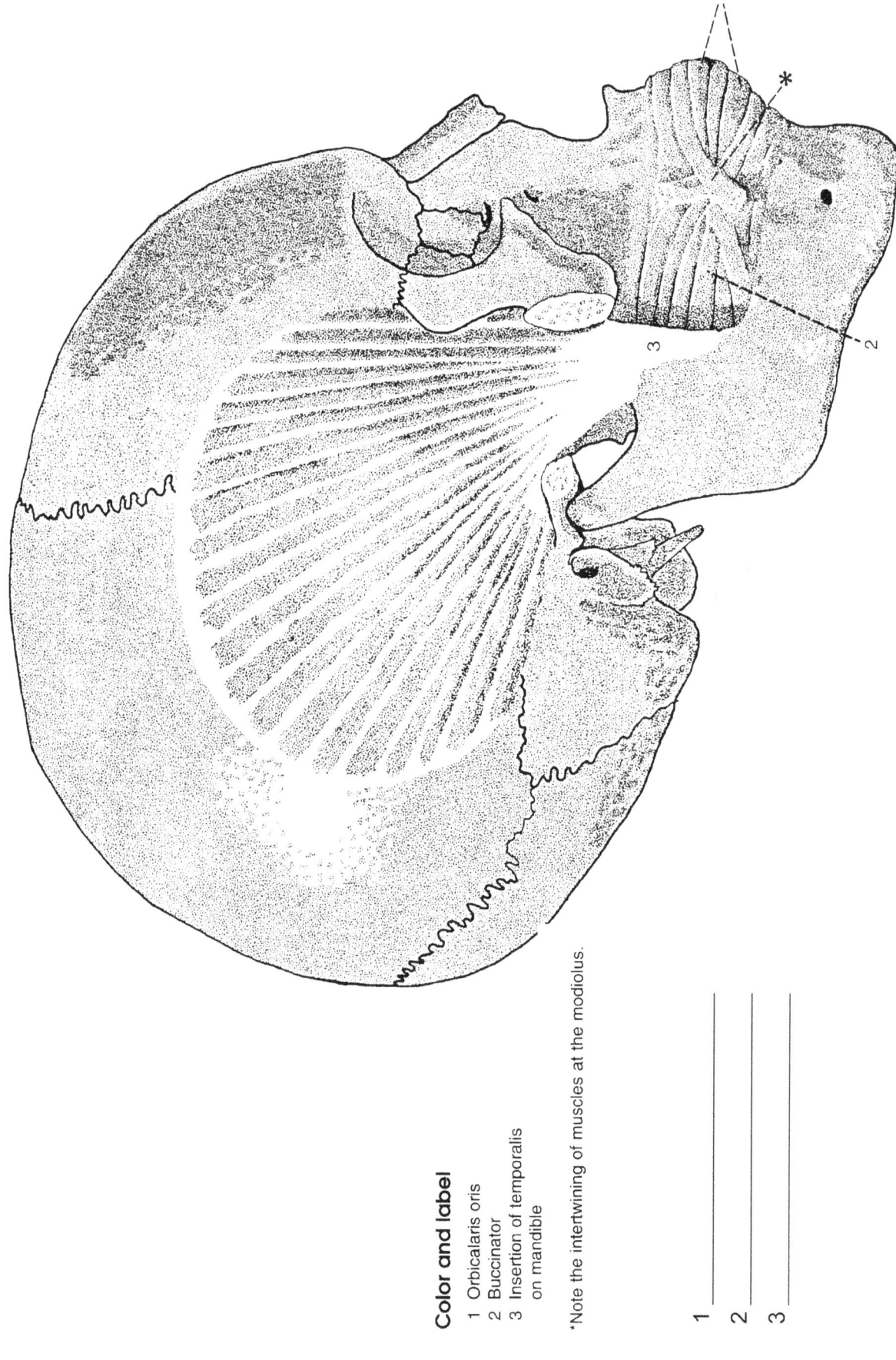

Color and label
1 Orbicalaris oris
2 Buccinator
3 Insertion of temporalis on mandible

*Note the intertwining of muscles at the modiolus.

1 _____
2 _____
3 _____

H&N-11 Median section of skull and mandible
Viewed from the left

Label these landmarks

1. Mandible and genial tubercle
2. Anterior nasal spine
3. Vomer
4. Perpindicular plate of ethmoid
5. Crista galli (Latin, cock's comb)
6. Optic canal
7. Anterior clinoid process
8. Squamous suture
9. Dorsum sellae
10. Groove for sigmoid sinus
11. Jugular foramen
12. Internal auditory meatus
13. Hypoglossal foramen
14. Sella turcica (Latin, Turkish saddle)
15. Sphenoid sinus
16. Lateral pterygoid plate (part of sphenoid bone)
17. Medial pterygoid plate (part of sphenoid bone)
18. Hypophyseal fossa (site of pituitary gland)

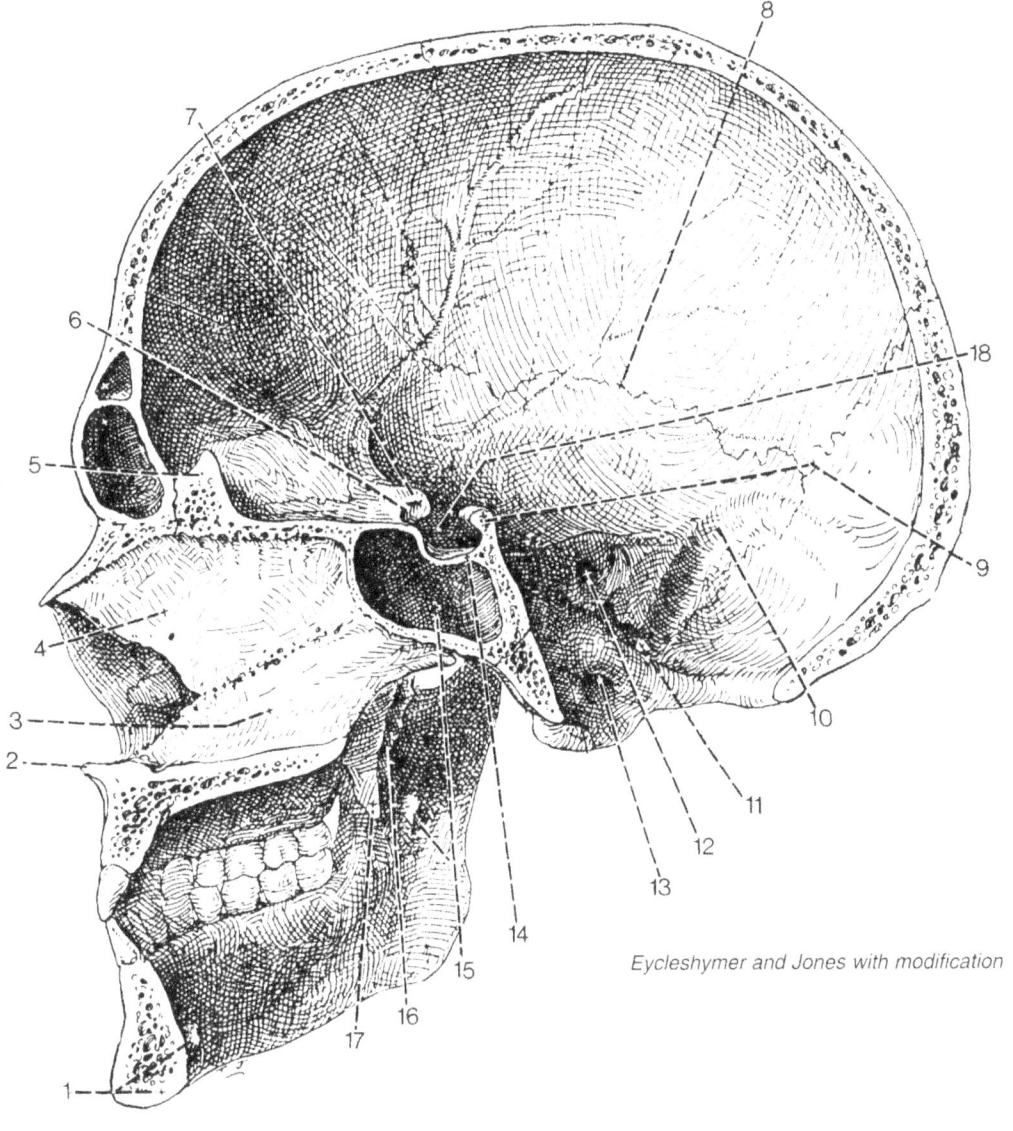

Eycleshymer and Jones with modification

1 _____
2 _____
3 _____
4 _____
5 _____
6 _____
7 _____
8 _____
9 _____
10 _____
11 _____
12 _____
13 _____
14 _____
15 _____
16 _____
17 _____
18 _____

H&N-12 Interior of the skull

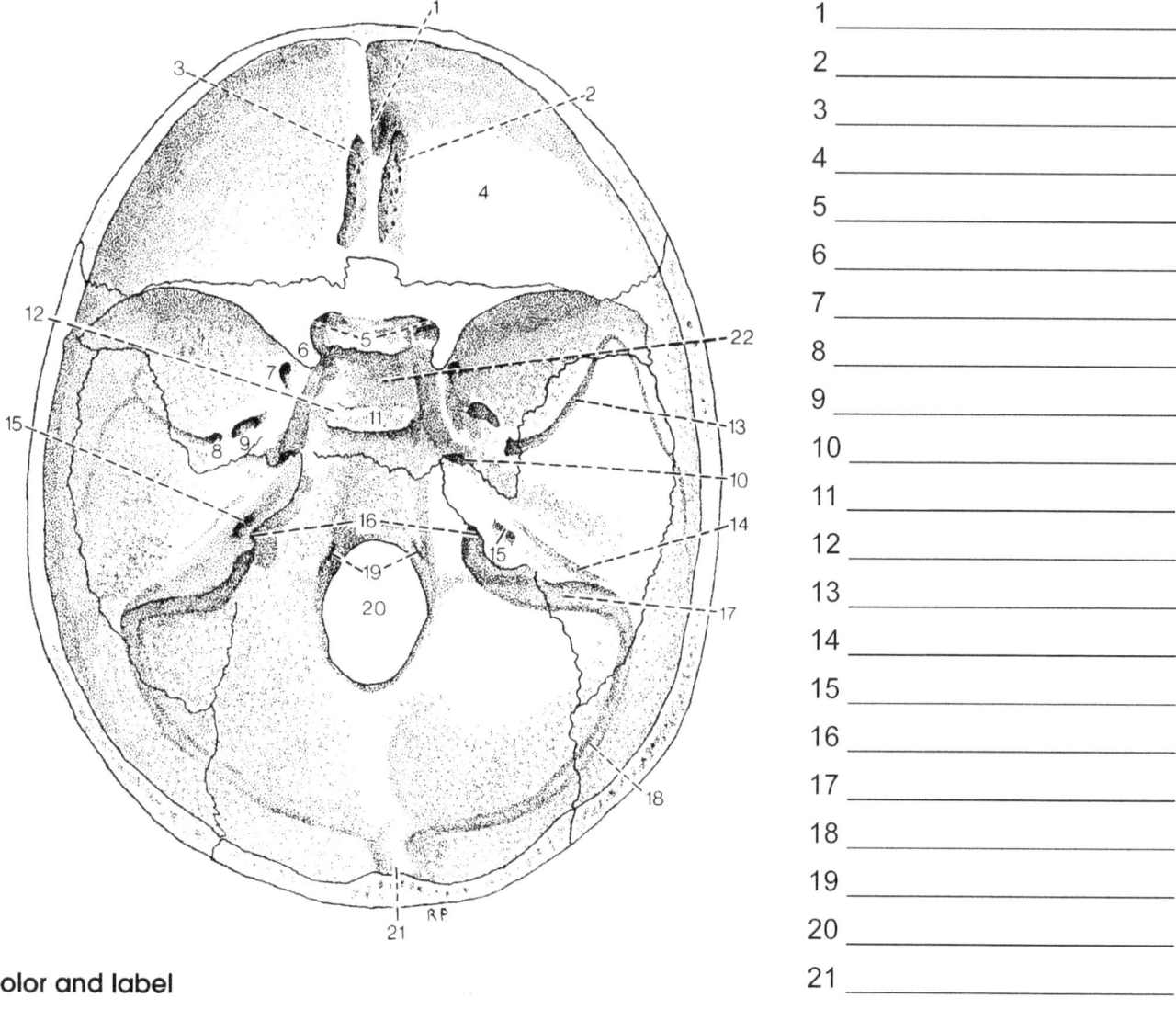

1. _____
2. _____
3. _____
4. _____
5. _____
6. _____
7. _____
8. _____
9. _____
10. _____
11. _____
12. _____
13. _____
14. _____
15. _____
16. _____
17. _____
18. _____
19. _____
20. _____
21. _____
22. _____

Color and label

1. Crista galli
2. Cribriform plate of ethmoid bone
3. Foramina for olfactory nerve fibers (cranial nerve I)
4. Orbital part of frontal bone
5. Optic canal; transmits optic nerve (cranial nerve II) and ophthalmic artery
6. Anterior clinoid process
7. Foramen rotundum (transmits maxillary branch of trigeminal nerve)
8. Foramen spinosum (transmits the middle meningeal artery and the meningeal branch of the mandibular nerve into the middle cranial fossa)
9. Foramen ovale (also called oval foramen of sphenoid bone; transmits mandibular branch of trigeminal nerve)
10. Foramen lacerum (in life it does not exit, rather it is filled with cartilage)
11. Dorsum sellae
12. Posterior clinoid process
13. Groove for middle meningeal artery
14. Groove for superior petrosal sinus*
15. Internal auditory meatus; passage conveying the facial nerve (cranial nerve VII), the vestibulocochlear nerve (cranial nerve VIII), and the labyrinthine artery
16. Jugular foramen; it transmits the glossopharyngeal nerve, the vagus nerve, the accessory nerve, and the internal jugular vein (continuation of the sigmoid sinus)
17. Sulcus for sigmoid sinus*
18. Sulcus for transverse sinus*
19. Hypoglossal canal
20. Foramen magnum
21. Sulcus for superior sagittal sinus*
22. Hypophyseal fossa (site of pituitary gland)

*These sinuses are dural venous sinuses that drain blood from the brain and bones of the cranium. They are located between two layers of dura mater, are lined with endothelium, and lack valves.

H&N-13 Superficial veins of the head and neck

Color and label

1. Superficial temporal vein
2. Middle temporal vein
3. Transverse facial vein
4. Maxillary vein (runs deep to mandible)
5. Retromandibular vein
6. Posterior auricular vein
7. External jugular vein
8. Anterior jugular vein
9. Posterior external jugular vein
10. Occipital vein
11. Facial vein
12. Submental vein
13. Inferior labial vein
14. Superior labial vein
15. Deep facial vein
16. Parotid ramus
17. External nasal vein
18. Inferior palpebral vein
19. Superior palpebral vein
20. Supratrochlear vein
21. Supraorbital vein
22. Internal jugular vein
23. Superior thyroid vein
24. Angular vein
25. Connection between angular vein and superior ophthalmic vei
26. Sternocleidomastoid muscle
27. Outline of parotid gland
28. Thyroid gland

Veins tend to vary in their pattern more than arteries and nerves.

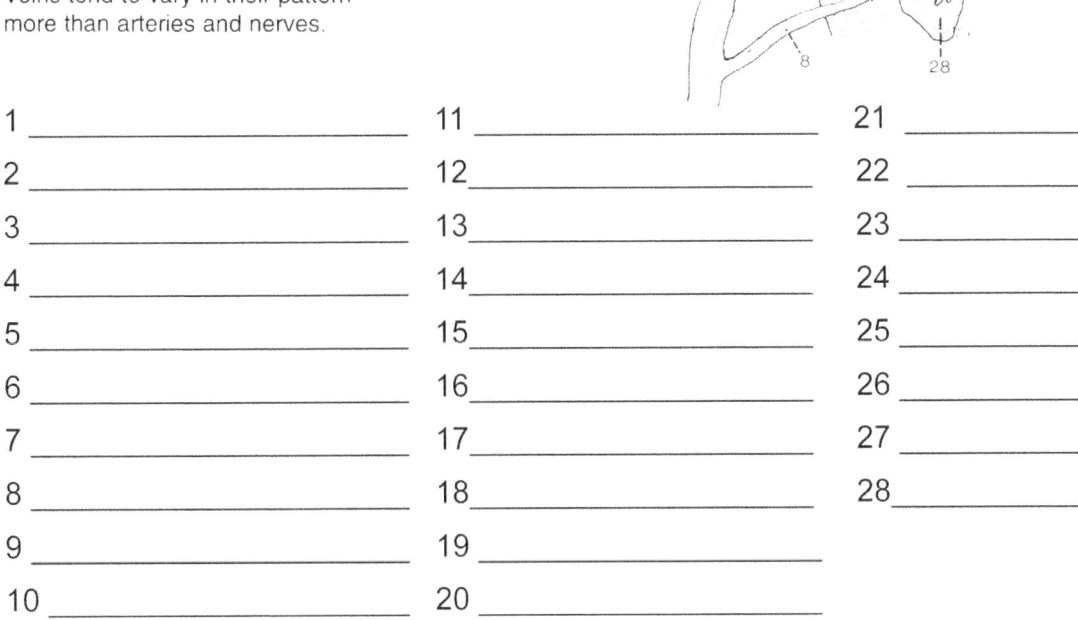

1 _____
2 _____
3 _____
4 _____
5 _____
6 _____
7 _____
8 _____
9 _____
10 _____
11 _____
12 _____
13 _____
14 _____
15 _____
16 _____
17 _____
18 _____
19 _____
20 _____
21 _____
22 _____
23 _____
24 _____
25 _____
26 _____
27 _____
28 _____

H&N-14 External carotid artery and its branches

Color and label
1. Common carotid artery
2. Internal carotid artery (gives off no branches until it enters the cranium)
3. External carotid artery
4. Superior thyroid artery
5. Ascending pharyngeal artery
6. Lingual artery
7. Facial artery
8. Occipital artery
9. Posterior auricular artery
10. Superficial temporal artery
11. Maxillary artery
12. Superior laryngeal artery
13. Submental artery
14. Inferior labial artery
15. Superior labial artery
16. Lateral nasal artery
17. Angular artery
18. Descending branch of occipital artery
19. Terminal branches of occipital artery
20. Transverse facial artery
21. Zygomatico-orbital artery
22. Frontal branch of superficial temporal artery
23. Parietal branch of superficial temporal artery
24. Middle meningeal artery
25. Inferior alveolar artery
26. Mylohyoid artery
27. Mental artery
28. Infraorbital artery
29. Posterior superior alveolar artery
30. Supraorbital artery
31. Supratrochlear artery

*Points of anastomoses

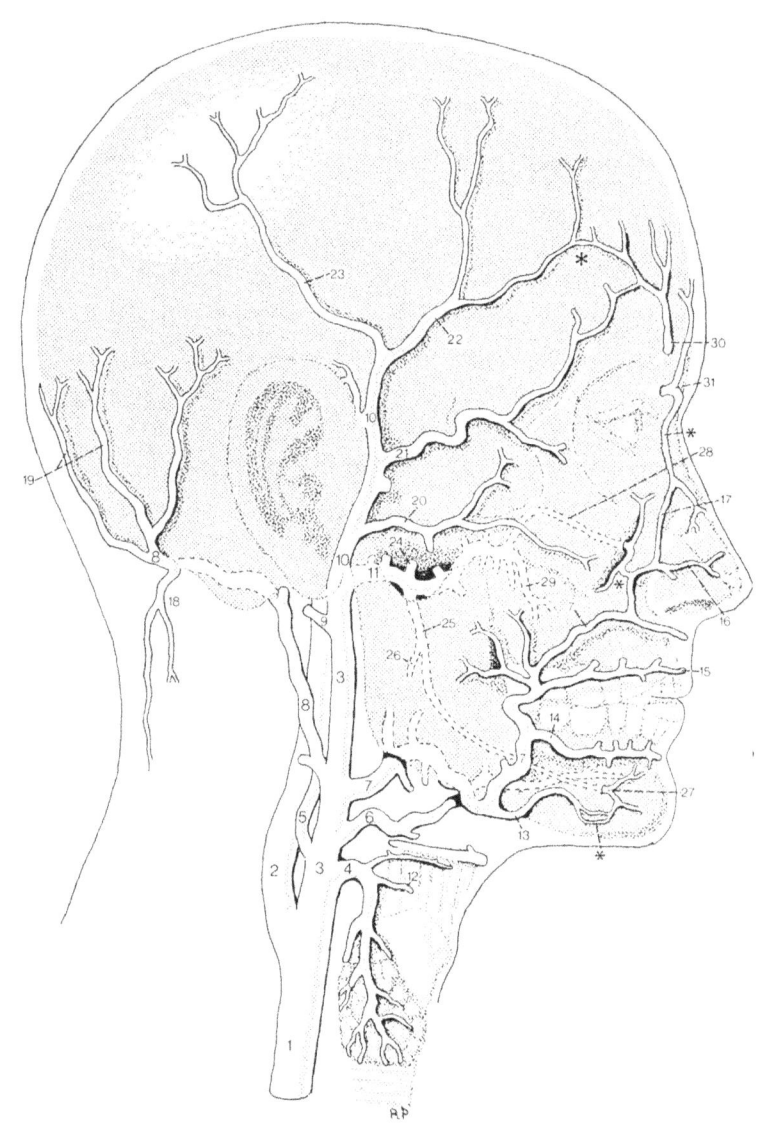

1. _____
2. _____
3. _____
4. _____
5. _____
6. _____
7. _____
8. _____
9. _____
10. _____
11. _____
12. _____
13. _____
14. _____
15. _____
16. _____
17. _____
18. _____
19. _____
20. _____
21. _____
22. _____
23. _____
24. _____
25. _____
26. _____
27. _____
28. _____
29. _____
30. _____
31. _____

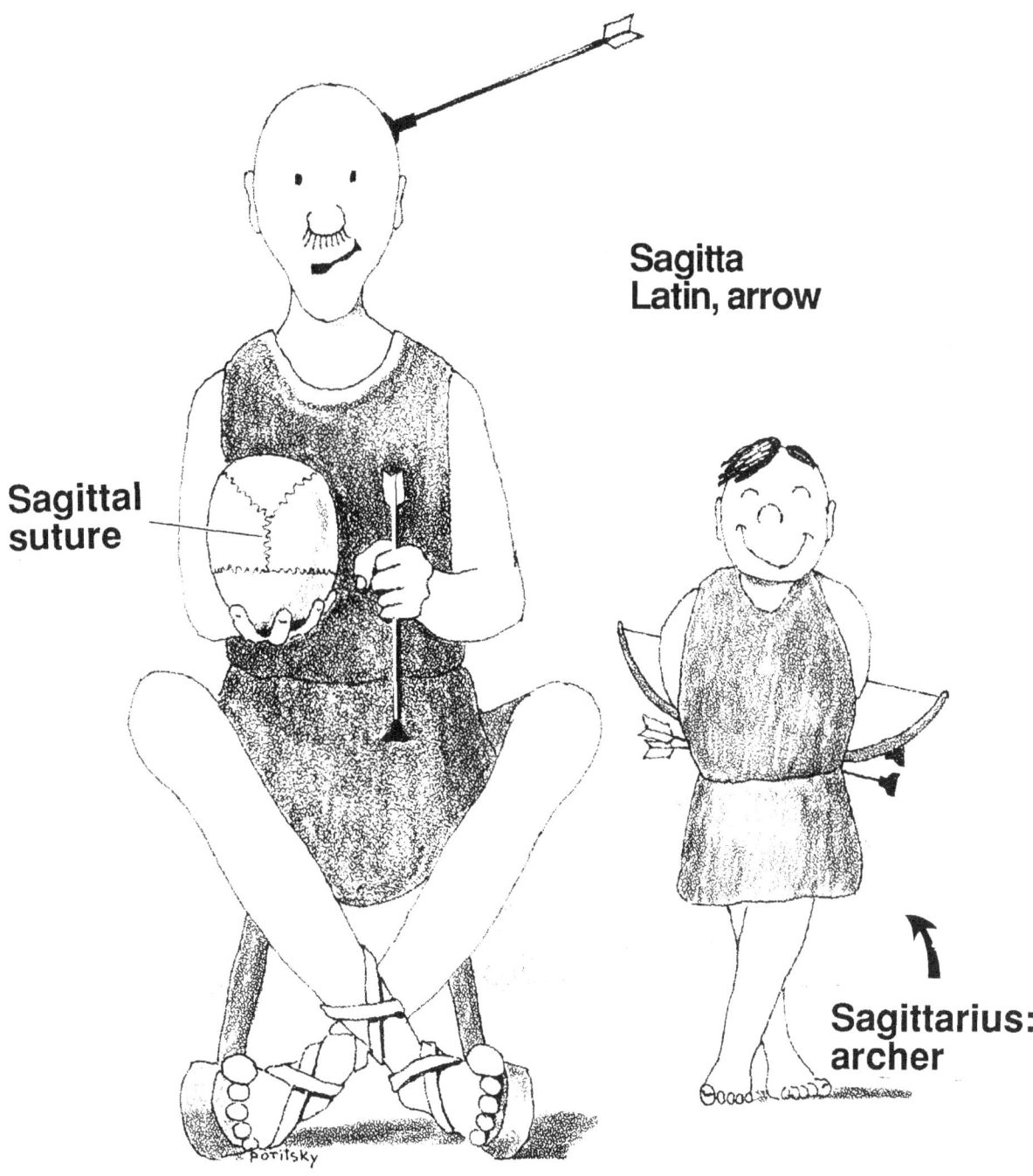

Sagitta is Latin for arrow. The sagittal plane in anatomy takes its name from the sagittal suture on the top of the skull, which runs between the two parietal bones in a front-to-back direction. At the back of the skull the sagittal suture meets the inverted V-shape of the lambdoid suture. With a bit of imagining one can visualize the sagittal suture forming the shaft of an arrow and a portion of the lambdoid forming the feathers.

H&N-15 Cranial dural venous sinuses

Beneath the brain

Color and label

1. Superior sagittal sinus (cut open)
2. Straight sinus (cut open)
3. Right transverse sinus (cut open)
4. Sigmoid sinus (cut open)
5. Occipital sinus
6. Confluence of sinuses
7. Cavernous sinus (cut open on left)
8. Superior petrosal sinus
9. Inferior petrosal sinus
10. Basilar venous plexus
11. Middle meningeal vein
12. Sphenoparietal sinus
13. Anterior and posterioir intercavernous sinuses
14. Superior ophthalmic vein
15. Tentorium cerebelli (cut and pulled to the right)
16. Pituitary gland (cut at stalk; also called hypophysis)

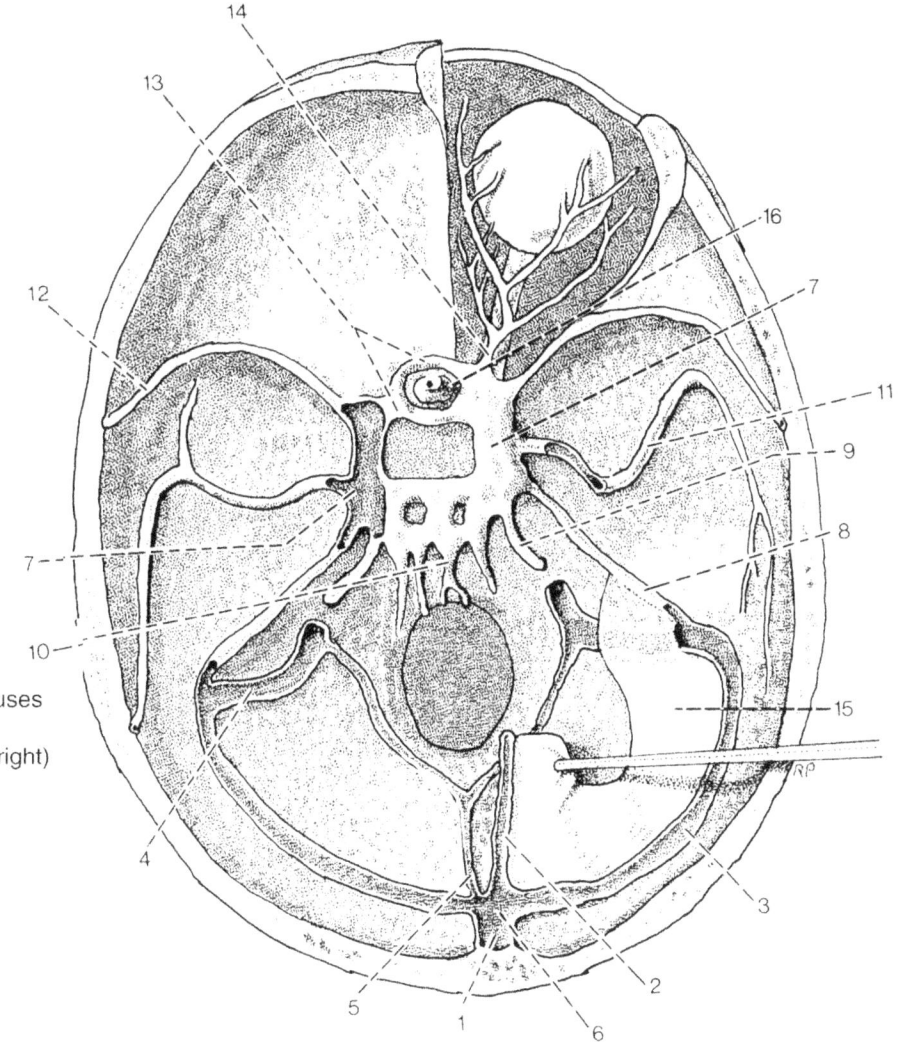

1 _____
2 _____
3 _____
4 _____
5 _____
6 _____
7 _____
8 _____
9 _____
10 _____
11 _____
12 _____
13 _____
14 _____
15 _____
16 _____

H&N-16 Head and neck

Midsagittal aspect

(opposite page)

Color and label

1. Scalp (skin and soft tissue covering the head that bears hair in both sexes)
2. Calavaria (the upper dome-like part of the skull or cranium, comprising the upper parts of the parietal, frontal and occipital bones)
3. Diploe (red bone marrow between the two layers of compact bone of the cranium)
4. Superior sagittal sinus (cut open to show opening of a superior cerebral vein)
5. Falx cerebri (a sickle-shaped fold of dura mater between the two cerebral hemispheres; *falx*, Latin, a sickle or scythe)
6. Inferior sagittal sinus
7. Crista galli (Latin, rooster's comb)
8. Straight sinus
9. Great cerebral vein
10. Confluence of sinuses
11. Opening of right transverse sinus
12. Occipital sinus
13. Falx cerebelli
14. Frontal sinus
15. Corpus callosum
16. Anterior cerebral artery
17. Septum pellucidum
18. Fornix
19. Thalamus and interthalamic adhesion
20. Optic chiasm
21. Pituitary gland (hypophysis)
22. Sphenoidal sinus
23. Mamillary body
24. Midbrain (mesencephalon)
25. Mesencephalic tectum
26. Pineal gland
27. Cerebral aqueduct
28. Cerebellum
29. Fourth ventricle
30. Cisternal magna (an enlargement of the subarachnoid space filled with cerebrospinal fluid under the cerebellum)
31. Basilar artery
32. Left vertebral artery
33. Pons
34. Medulla oblongata
35. Spinal cord
36. Anterior arch of atlas
37. Body and dens of atlas
38. Pharyngeal tonsil
39. Opening of auditory tube (eustachian tube)
40. Nasal pharynx
41. Middle nasa concha
42. Inferior nasal concha
43. Hard palate
44. Soft palate and uvula
45. Mandible
46. Hyoid bone
47. Genioglossus muscle
48. Geniohyoid muscle
49. Mylohyoid muscle
50. Epiglottis
51. Thyroid cartilage
52. Cricoid cartilage (arch and lamina)
53. Trachea
54. Oral pharynx
55. Laryngeal pharynx
56. Esophagus

1 _____
2 _____
3 _____
4 _____
5 _____
6 _____
7 _____
8 _____
9 _____
10 _____
11 _____
12 _____
13 _____
14 _____
15 _____
16 _____
17 _____
18 _____
19 _____
20 _____
21 _____
22 _____
23 _____
24 _____
25 _____
26 _____
27 _____
28 _____
29 _____
30 _____

H&N-16 Head and neck
Midsagittal aspect

31 _____
32 _____
33 _____
34 _____
35 _____
36 _____
37 _____
38 _____
39 _____
40 _____
41 _____
42 _____
43 _____
44 _____
45 _____
46 _____
47 _____
48 _____
49 _____
50 _____
51 _____
52 _____
53 _____
54 _____
55 _____
56 _____

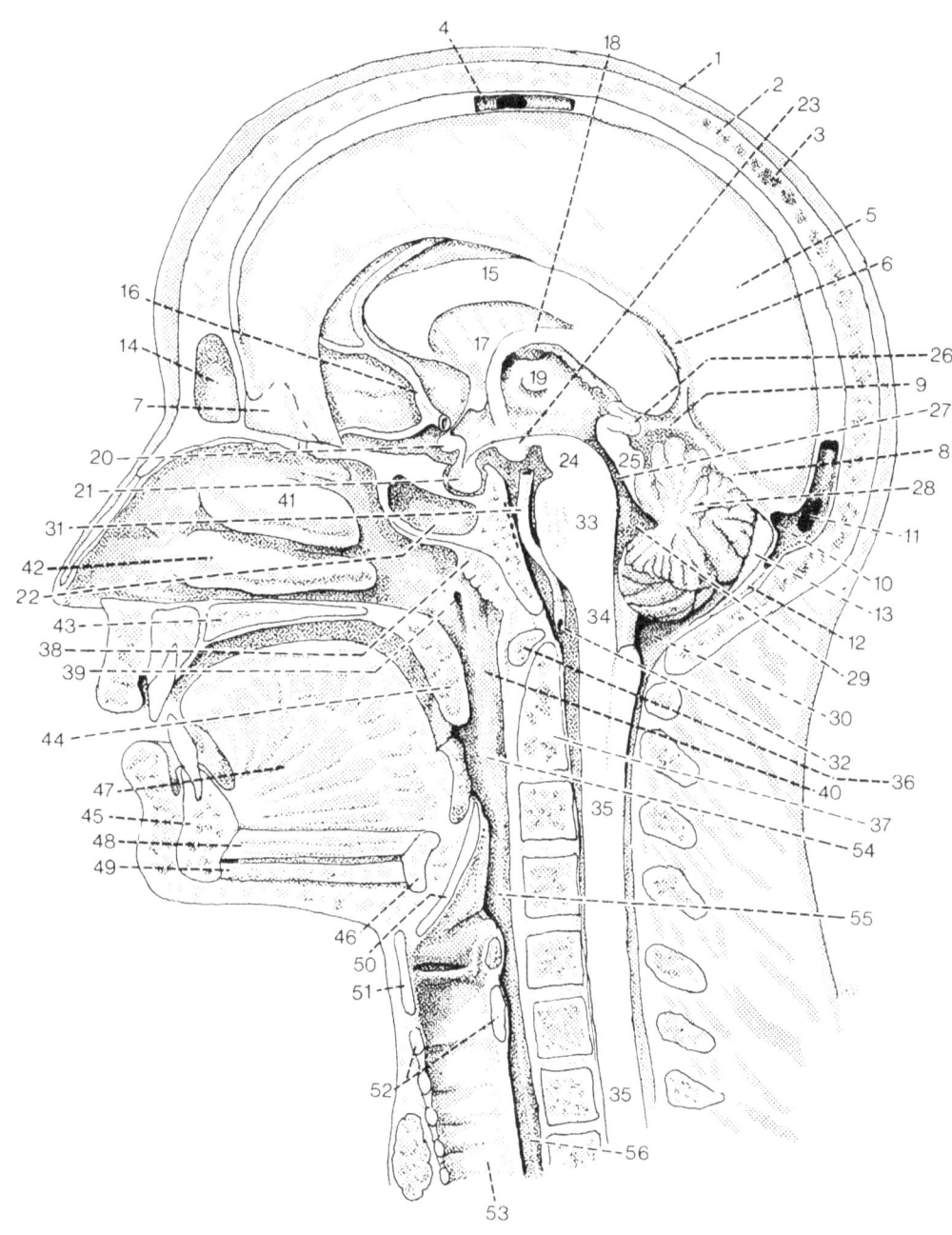

H&N-17 Superior sagittal sinus

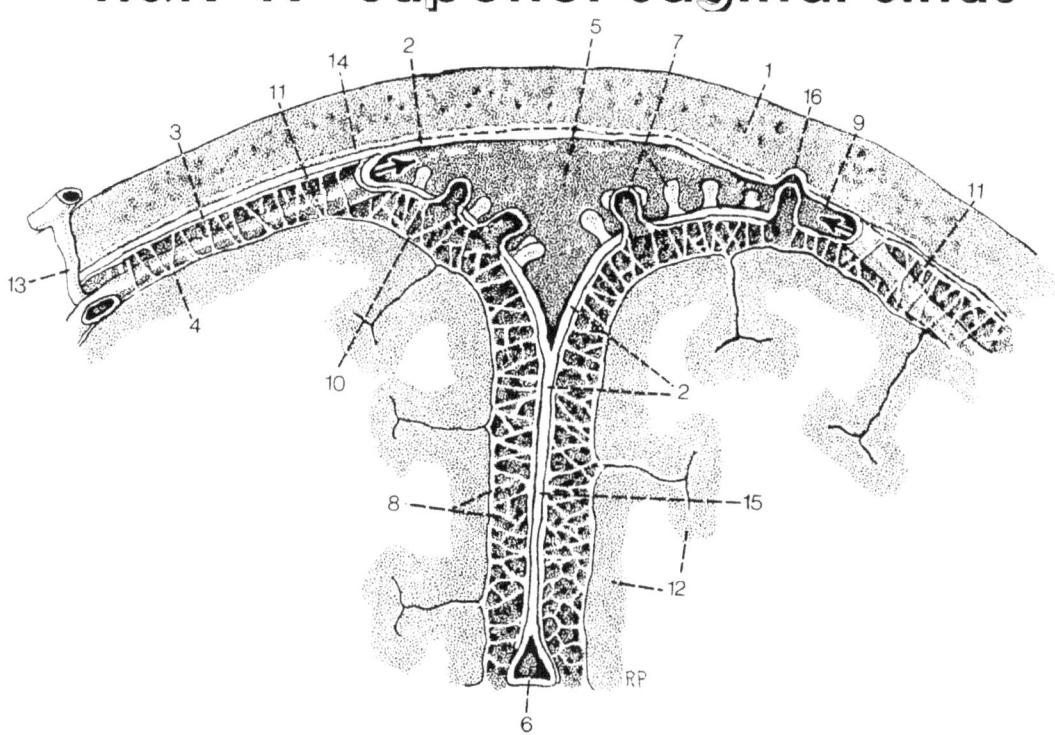

Color and labe

1. Bone of skull
2. Dura mater (tough outermost membrane covering the brain and spinal cord)
3. Arachnoid (also called arachnoid membrane); closely applied to the inner surface of the dura mater; middle covering membrane (or meninx, plural, meninges)
4. Pia mater (innermost membrance investing the brain and spinal cord)
5. Superior sagittal sinus (large arched vein; drains blood from the brain, formed by walls of dura mater).
6. Inferior sagittal sinus
7. Arachnoid granulations; hollow finger-like projections into the superior sagittal sinus and its lateral expansions; these contain cerebrospinal fluid from the subarachnoid space which drains into and mixes with the venous blood of the superior sagittal sinus.
8. Arachnoid trabeculae; these form a mesh-work of small fibers that crisscross the subarachnoid space.
9. Lateral lacunae (outpouchings of the superior sagittal sinus)
10. Subarachnoid space (present between arachnoid and pia mater contains cerebrospinal fluid)
11. Superior cerebral vein emptying into superior sagittal sinus
12. Cerebral cortex
13. Emissary vein; these pass completely through the skull; link intracranial venous blood flow with external veins.
14. Periosteum of skull
15. Falx cerebri (*falx*, Latin, a sickle or scythe)
16. Pit on inside of skull caused by arachnoid granulation

1 _____
2 _____
3 _____
4 _____
5 _____
6 _____
7 _____
8 _____
9 _____
10 _____
11 _____
12 _____
13 _____
14 _____
15 _____
16 _____

H&N-18 Interior of the skull with cranial nerve exits
(OPPOSITE PAGE)

Color and label

1. Optic nerve (cranial nerve II) exiting skull through optic canal
2. Internal carotid artery
3. Ophthalmic artery arising from internal carotid
4. Trigeminal ganglion
5. Sensory root of trigeminal nerve
6. Motor root of trigeminal nerve
7. Oculomotor nerve (cranial nerve III)
8. Trochlear nerve (cranial nerve IV)
9. Abducent nerve (cranial nerve VI)
10. Pituitary gland (*pituita*, Latin, phlegm)*
11. Cut edge of dura mater
12. Ophthalmic nerve
13. Frontal nerve
14. Nasocilliary nerve
15. Lacrimal nerve
16. Supraorbital nerve
17. Supratrochlear nerve
18. Maxillary nerve
19. Mandibular nerve
20. Middle meningeal artery entering skull
21. Facial nerve motor root (cranial nerve VII)
22. Nervus intermedius of facial nerve (cranial nerve VII)
23. Vestibulocochlear nerve (cranial nerve VIII)
24. Glossopharyngeal nerve (cranial nerve IX)
25. Vagus nerve (cranial nerve X)
26. Accessory nerve (cranial nerve XI)
27. Hypoglossal nerve (cranial nerve XII)
28. Vertebral artery (right and left)
29. Internal acoustic meatus
30. Jugular foramen
31. Hypoglossal canal
32. Roof of orbit (cut and removed)
33. Roof of orbit
34. Cribriform plate (of ethmoid bone) with foramina for about 20 olfactory fila; each filum contains bundles of unmyelinated olfactory axons from olfactory receptors in the roof of the nasal cavity; the olfactory fila (not shown) collectively make up the olfactory nerve (cranial nerve I)

* See cartoon. Thalamus means bedroom.

1 _____
2 _____
3 _____
4 _____
5 _____
6 _____
7 _____
8 _____
9 _____
10 _____
11 _____
12 _____
13 _____
14 _____
15 _____
16 _____
17 _____
18 _____
19 _____
20 _____
21 _____
22 _____
23 _____
24 _____
25 _____
26 _____
27 _____
28 _____
29 _____
30 _____
31 _____
32 _____
33 _____
34 _____

H&N-18 Interior of the skull with cranial nerve exits

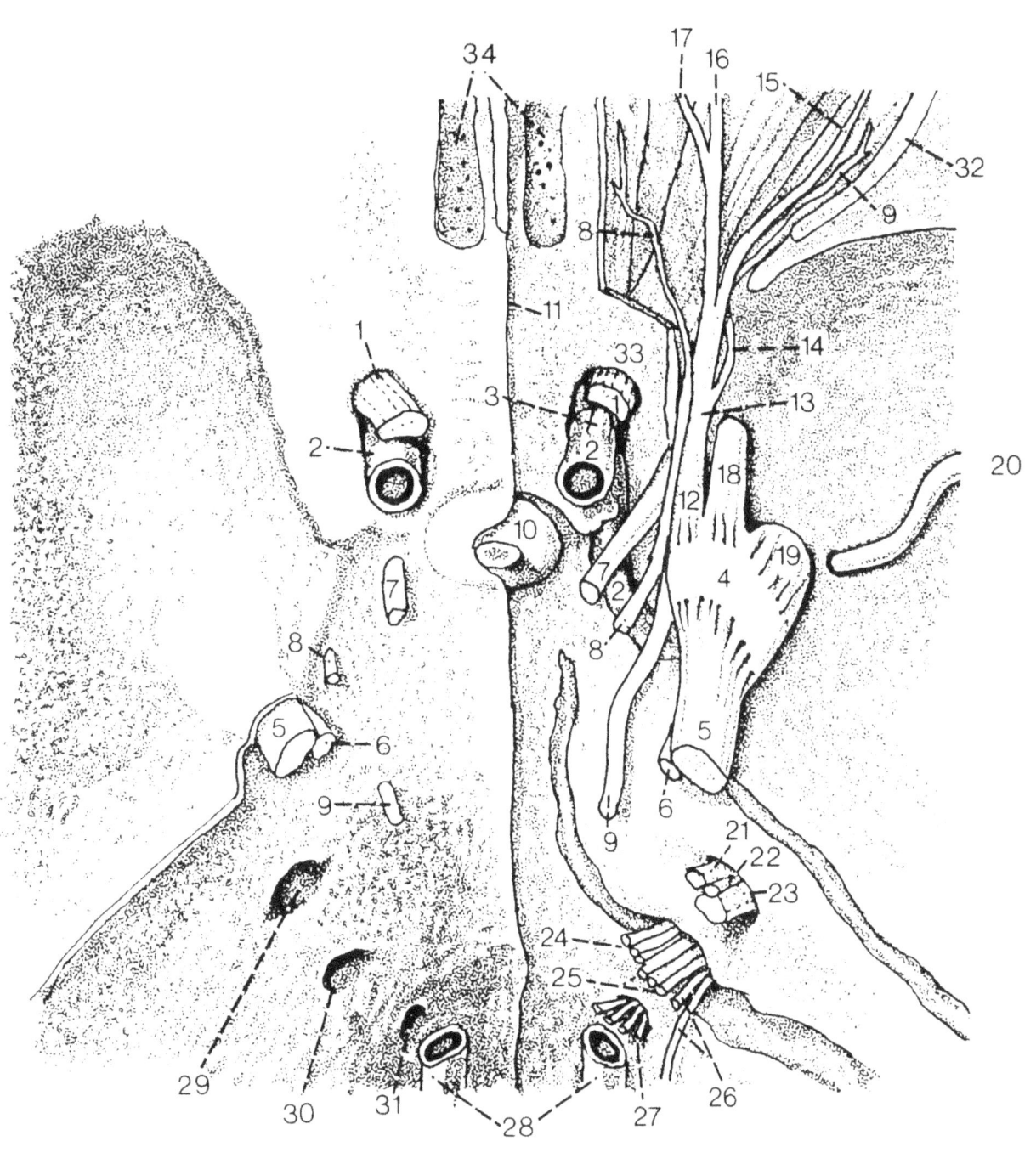

H&N-19 Facial nerve and its branches

Color and label

1. Facial nerve; here lying in the internal auditory meatus accompanied by the vestibulocochlear nerve (not shown) and internal auditory vessels (not shown); taste fibers and parasympathetic fibers travel in the nervus intermedius part of the facial nerve.
2. Geniculate ganglion (contains nerve cell bodies of taste fibers to anterior two-thirds of tongue and some general sensory fibers to the skin of the external ear)
3. Greater petrosal nerve (carries taste fibers to the palate and preganglionic parasympathetic fibers, which synapse in the pterygopalatine ganglion)
4. Chorda tympani nerve; this nerve leaves the facial nerve in its descending part of the facial canal, enters the tympanic cavity, crosses the upper part of the internal surface of the tympanic membrane (hence its name), leaves the skull through the petrotympanic fissure, joins the lingual nerve, and supplies the taste buds on the anterior two-thirds of the tongue. Its preganglionic parasympathetic fibers synapse in the submandibular ganglion.
5. Nerve to stapedius muscle (damage to the facial nerve proximal to this branch will cause stapedius to lose its damping action and sounds will be unusually loud)
6. Lingual nerve (cut; part of the mandibular nerve)
7. Deep petrosal nerve (postganglionic sympathetic fibers from the internal carotid plexus)
8. Nerve of pterygoid canal (note that it consists of the deep petrosal nerve and the greater petrosal nerve)
9. Pterygopalatine ganglion (contains postganglionic parasympathetic neurons whose secretomotor fibers enter the nasal cavity and supply glands and vessels in the nose)
10. Internal carotid plexus (sympathetic nerve fibers from cell bodies in the superior cervical ganglion)
11. Submandibular ganglion (sends postganglionic secretomotor fibers to the submandibular gland and sublingual salivary glands)
12. Maxillary nerve (cut; exiting skull via foramen rotundum)
13. Infraorbital nerve
14. Posterior superior alveolar nerve (to posterior superior teeth)
15. Palatine nerves (descend to supply palate)
16. Pterygopalatine nerves (convey postganglionic parasympathetic secretomotor fibers from ganglion to maxillary nerve to zygomatic nerve to lacrimal nerve to lacrimal gland)
17. Middle superior alveolar nerve (to superior teeth)
18. Zygomatic nerve
19. Communicating branch to lacrimal nerve
20. Lacrimal nerve
21. Internal carotid artery
22. Mastoid process
23. Styloid process
24. Ear drum and malleus
25. Stylomastoid foramen
26. Facial canal
27. Carotid canal
28. Foramen lacerum
29. Medial pterygoid plate
30. Canal and groove for greater petrosal nerve
31. Orbit (eye and muscles removed)
32. Internal acoustic meatus (roof removed)

(Use abbrevs.)

1 _____
2 _____
3 _____
4 _____
5 _____
6 _____
7 _____
8 _____
9 _____
10 _____
11 _____
12 _____
13 _____
14 _____
15 _____
16 _____
17 _____
18 _____
19 _____
20 _____
21 _____
22 _____
23 _____
24 _____
25 _____
26 _____
27 _____
28 _____
29 _____
30 _____
31 _____
32 _____

H&N-19 Facial nerve and its branches

Lateral view of facial nerve with internal auditory meatus and canal exposed, carotid canal opened, and greater wing of sphenoid removed

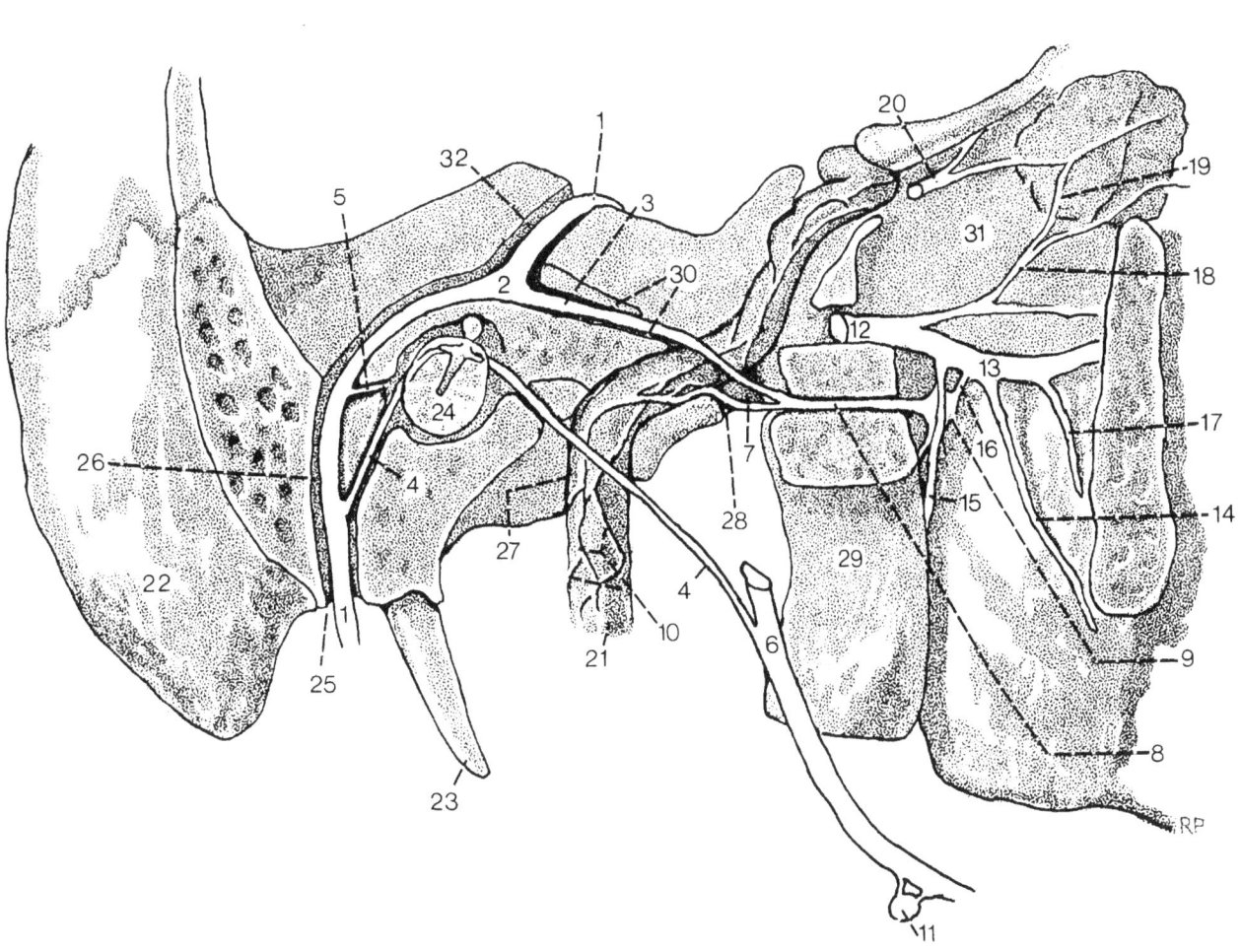

H&N-20 Functional components of the facial nerve

(opposite page)

Color and label these nerve cells and their fibers (axons)

1. Motor neuron to muscles of facial expression (also to platysma, stapedius, stylohyoid, and posterior belly of digastric)
2. Facial motor nucleus
3. Parasympathetic neuron (preganglionic secretomotor) to submandibular ganglion
4. Parasympathetic neuron (preganglionic secretomotor) to pterygopalatine ganglion
5. Superior salivatory ganglion
6. Cell body of neuron carrying taste from the tongue via chorda tympani nerve; note this neuron resides in the geniculate, or "bent", (*genu*, Latin, knee) ganglion of the facial nerve
7. Cell body of neuron carrying taste from the palate via the greater petrosal nerve
8. Neuron in nucleus of solitary tract; this neuron receives taste from incoming neuron taste fiber of neuron 6 and relays it to higher centers (not shown)
9. Neuron in nucleus of solitary tract; this neuron receives taste from incoming neuron taste fiber of neuron 7 and relays it to higher centers (not shown)
10. Nucleus of solitary tract
11. Parasympathetic neuron (postganglionic) in pterygopalatine ganglion secretomotor to lacrimal gland
12. Parasympathetic neuron (postganglionic) in pterygopalatine ganglion secretomotor to nasal glands
13. Pterygopalatine ganglion
14. Parasympathetic neuron (postganglionic) in submandibular ganglion secretomotor to submandibular gland
15. Parasympathetic neuron (postganglionic) in submandibular ganglion secretomotor to sublingual gland
16. Sympathetic neuron (preganglionic) in spinal cord
17. Sympathetic neuron (postganglionic) in superior cervial ganglion
18. Superior cervical ganglion
19. Internal carotid plexus
20. Geniculate ganglion of facial nerve
21. Greater petrosal nerve; note it carries both taste and parasympathetic fibers (parasympathetic root of pterygopalatine ganglion)
22. Deep petrosal nerve
23. Nerve of pterygoid canal; note it consists of taste fibers from the palate (neuron 9), parasympathetic fibers to the palate (neuron 4), and sympathetic fibers (fibers 22) to blood vessels and glands in the nose.
24. Nerve to tiny stapedius muscle in middle ear
25. Chorda tympani; note this nerve is a branch of the intermediate nerve of the facial nerve. It carries incoming taste from the tongue (neuron 6) and outgoing parasympathetic fibers to the submandibular gangion (neuron 3). In this sense, the chorda tympani nerve functions as the parasympathetic root of submandibular ganglion.
26. Facial canal
27. Stylomastoid foramen
28. Maxillary nerve in foramen rotundum (a small portion)
29. Lacrimal nerve (a branch of the ophthalmic nerve); it recieves its parasympathetic secretomotor fibers from nerve 11 in the pterygopalatine ganglion
30. Zygomatic nerve
31. Zygomaticotemporal nerve
32. Communicating branch between zygomaticotemporal nerve and lacrimal nerve
33. Facial nerve exiting stylomastoid foramen
34. Genu (or geniculum) "bend" or "knee" of facial nerve
35. Submandibular ganglion

Each nerve cell (or neuron) diagramatically represents hundred or even thousands of similarly directed neurons.

A **nucleus** is a group of nerve cells in the brain or spinal cord. A similar collection of neurons outside the brain and spinal cord is called **ganglion.**

H&N-20 Functional components of the facial nerve

(use abbrevs.)

1. _____
2. _____
3. _____
4. _____
5. _____
6. _____
7. _____
8. _____
9. _____
10. _____
11. _____
12. _____
13. _____
14. _____
15. _____
16. _____
17. _____
18. _____
19. _____
20. _____
21. _____
22. _____
23. _____
24. _____
25. _____
26. _____
27. _____
28. _____
29. _____
30. _____
31. _____
32. _____
33. _____
34. _____
35. _____

H&N-21 Inferior surface of skull

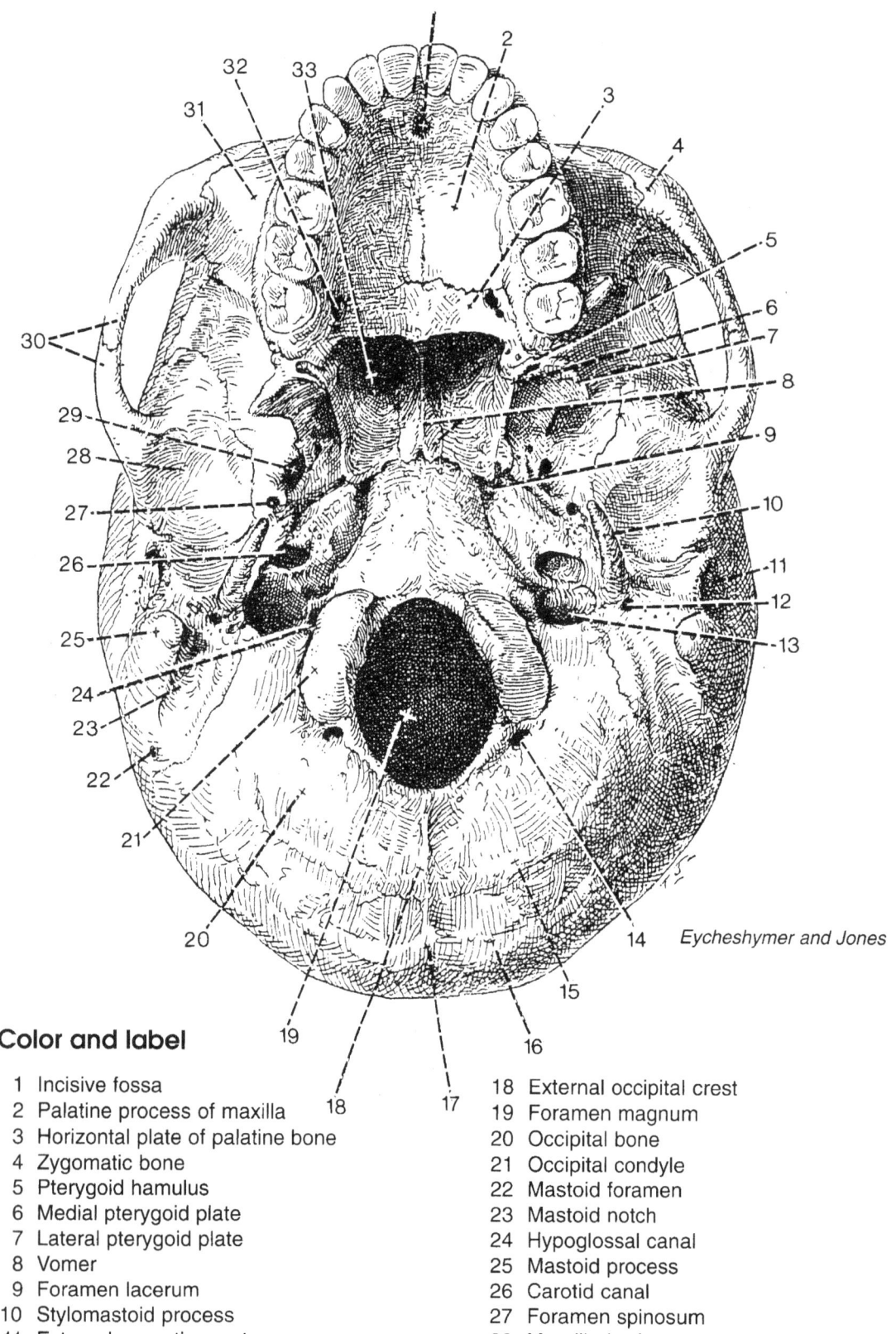

Eycheshymer and Jones

Color and label

1. Incisive fossa
2. Palatine process of maxilla
3. Horizontal plate of palatine bone
4. Zygomatic bone
5. Pterygoid hamulus
6. Medial pterygoid plate
7. Lateral pterygoid plate
8. Vomer
9. Foramen lacerum
10. Stylomastoid process
11. External acoustic meatus
12. Stylomastoid foramen
13. Jugular foramen
14. Condylar foramen
15. Inferior nuchal line
16. Superior nuchal line
17. External occipital protuberance
18. External occipital crest
19. Foramen magnum
20. Occipital bone
21. Occipital condyle
22. Mastoid foramen
23. Mastoid notch
24. Hypoglossal canal
25. Mastoid process
26. Carotid canal
27. Foramen spinosum
28. Mandibular fossa
29. Foramen ovale
30. Zygomatic arch
31. Maxilla
32. Greater and lesser palatine foramina
33. Posterior nasal aperature (choana)

(opposite page)

1 _____
2 _____
3 _____
4 _____
5 _____
6 _____
7 _____
8 _____
9 _____
10 _____
11 _____
12 _____
13 _____
14 _____
15 _____
16 _____
17 _____
18 _____
19 _____
20 _____
21 _____
22 _____
23 _____
24 _____
25 _____
26 _____
27 _____
28 _____
29 _____
30 _____
31 _____
32 _____
33 _____

Temporal
Etymological cartoon

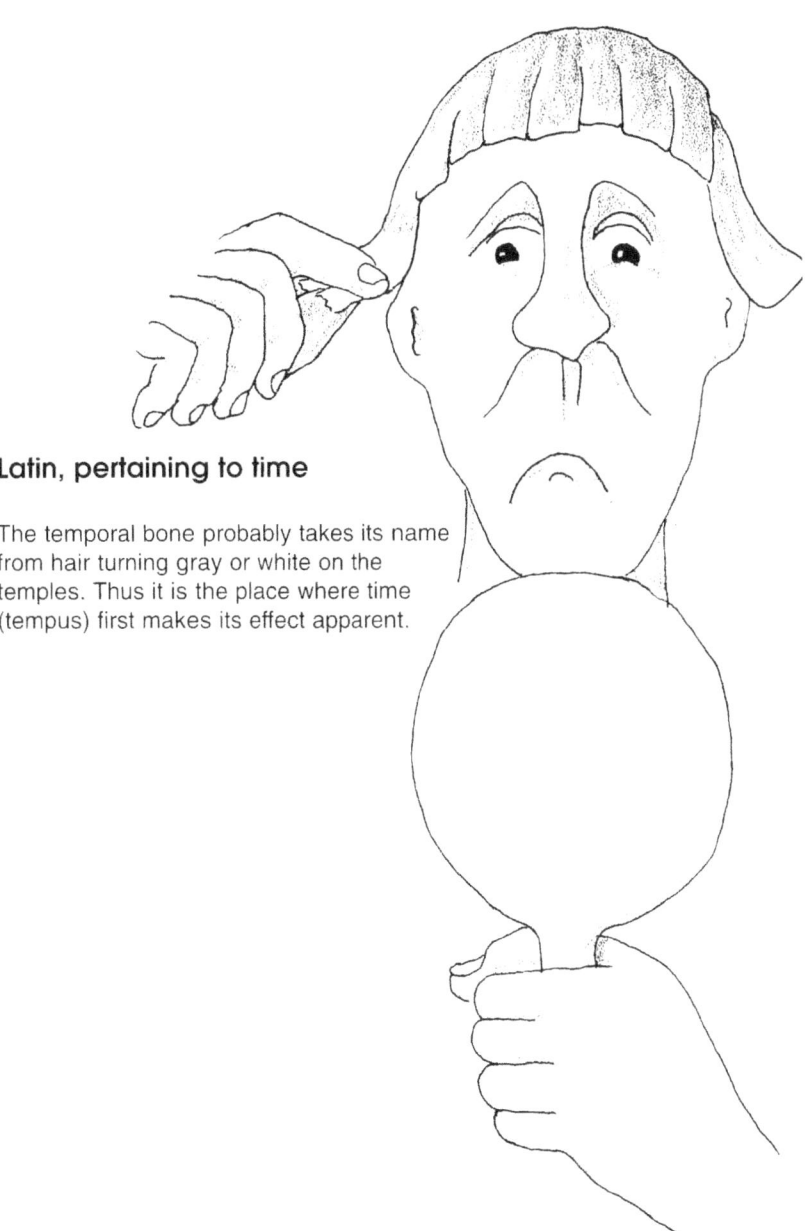

Latin, pertaining to time

The temporal bone probably takes its name from hair turning gray or white on the temples. Thus it is the place where time (tempus) first makes its effect apparent.

H&N-22 Sphenoid bone

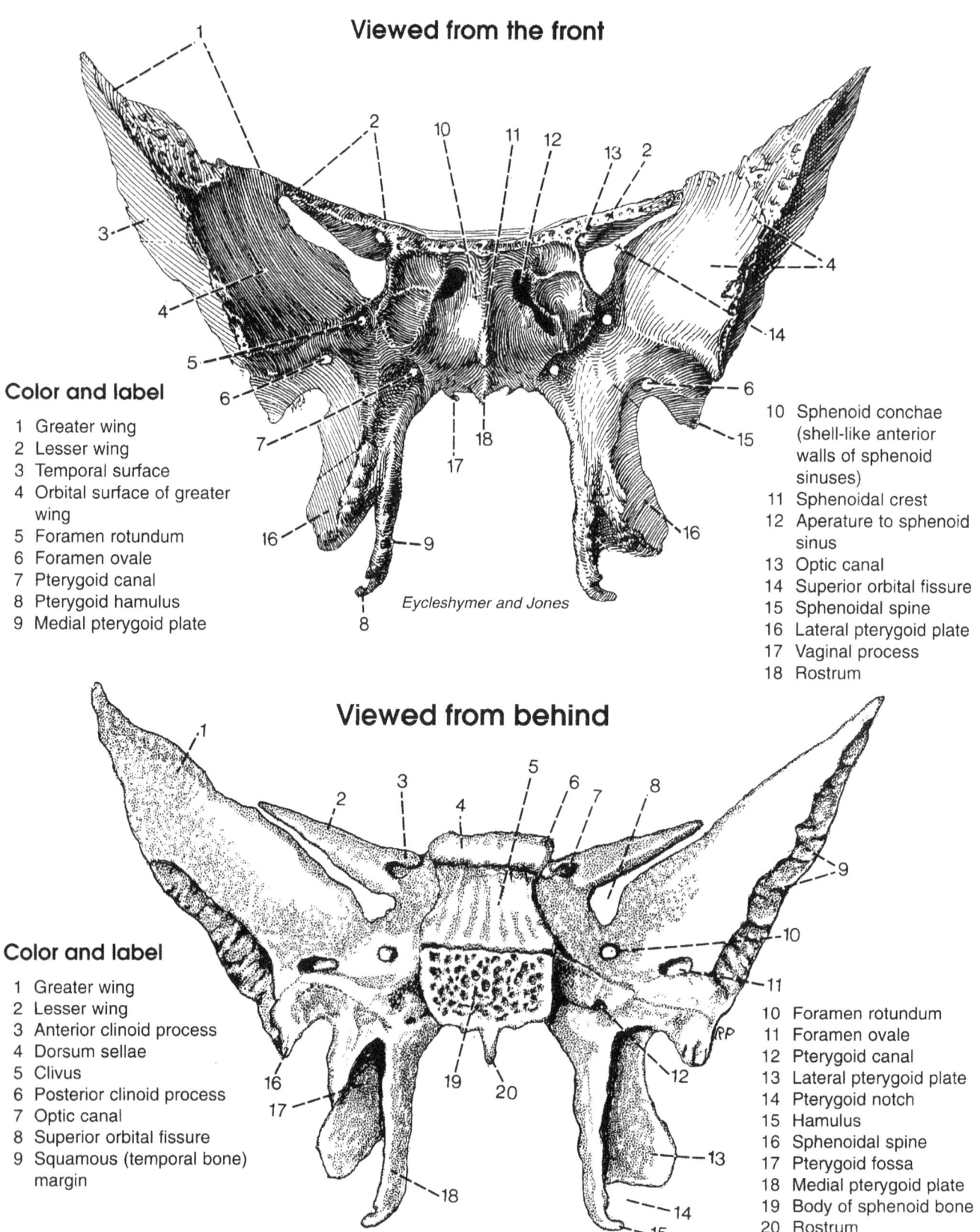

Viewed from the front

Color and label

1. Greater wing
2. Lesser wing
3. Temporal surface
4. Orbital surface of greater wing
5. Foramen rotundum
6. Foramen ovale
7. Pterygoid canal
8. Pterygoid hamulus
9. Medial pterygoid plate
10. Sphenoid conchae (shell-like anterior walls of sphenoid sinuses)
11. Sphenoidal crest
12. Aperature to sphenoid sinus
13. Optic canal
14. Superior orbital fissure
15. Sphenoidal spine
16. Lateral pterygoid plate
17. Vaginal process
18. Rostrum

Viewed from behind

Color and label

1. Greater wing
2. Lesser wing
3. Anterior clinoid process
4. Dorsum sellae
5. Clivus
6. Posterior clinoid process
7. Optic canal
8. Superior orbital fissure
9. Squamous (temporal bone) margin
10. Foramen rotundum
11. Foramen ovale
12. Pterygoid canal
13. Lateral pterygoid plate
14. Pterygoid notch
15. Hamulus
16. Sphenoidal spine
17. Pterygoid fossa
18. Medial pterygoid plate
19. Body of sphenoid bone
20. Rostrum

H&N-22 Sphenoid bone

Viewed from the front

1 _____
2 _____
3 _____
4 _____
5 _____
6 _____
7 _____
8 _____
9 _____

10 _____
11 _____
12 _____
13 _____
14 _____
15 _____
16 _____
17 _____
18 _____

Viewed from behind

1 _____
2 _____
3 _____
4 _____
5 _____
6 _____
7 _____
8 _____
9 _____
10 _____

11 _____
12 _____
13 _____
14 _____
15 _____
16 _____
17 _____
18 _____
19 _____
20 _____

H&N-23 Temporal bone

External surface viewed from the right

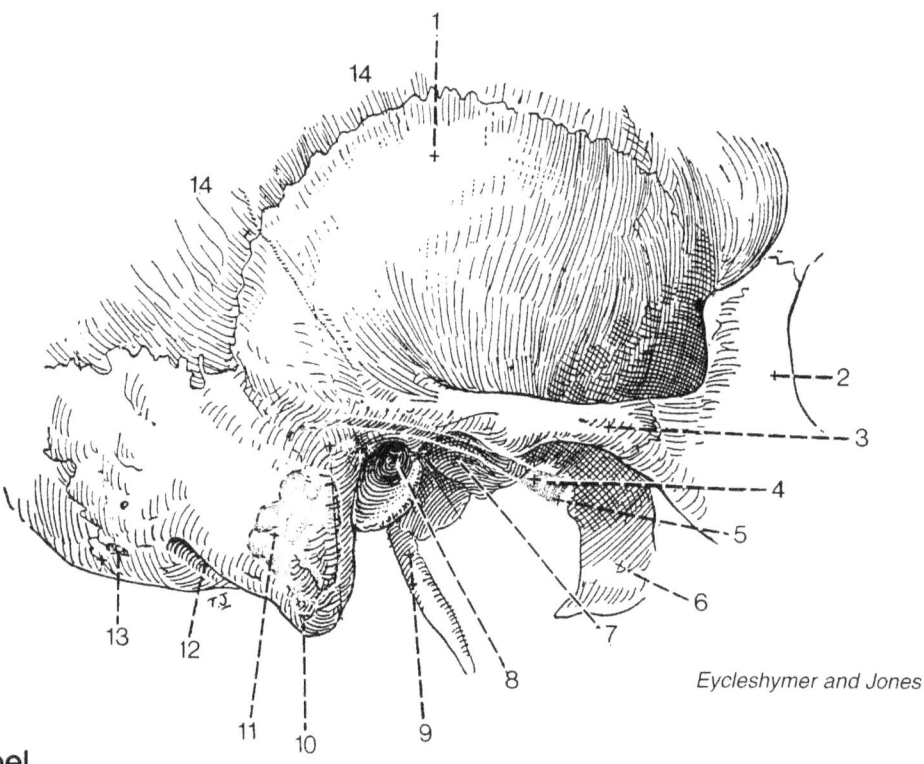

Eycleshymer and Jones

Color and label

1. Squamous part (scale-like, flat, and thin; *squama*, Latin, scale)
2. Zygomatic bone
3. Zygomatic process of temporal bone
4. Auditory tube (eustachian tube, cartilaginous part; this tube connects the middle ear with the nasopharynx; when temporarily opened it equalizes air pressure in the middle ear with the ambient air pressure)
5. Pharyngeal ostium (mouth) of auditory tube
6. Lateral pterygoid plate
7. Mandibular fossa (articulates with head of mandible; forms temporomandibular joint)
8. External acoustic meatus (bony part of ear canal)
9. Styloid process
10. Mastoid (breast-like, *mastos*, Greek, breast)
11. Mastoid air cells inside mastoid process (before antibiotics, infection of these air sinuses could be treated only by surgically scraping out most of the mastoid process air cells.
12. Mastoid notch (posterior belly of digastric muscle attaches to ridge; occipital artery lies in groove)
13. Mastoid foramen (through which passes an emissary vein)
14. Parietal bone

1 _____
2 _____
3 _____
4 _____
5 _____
6 _____
7 _____
8 _____
9 _____
10 _____
11 _____
12 _____
13 _____
14 _____

H&N-24 Temporal bone

Right bone. Viewed from the inside

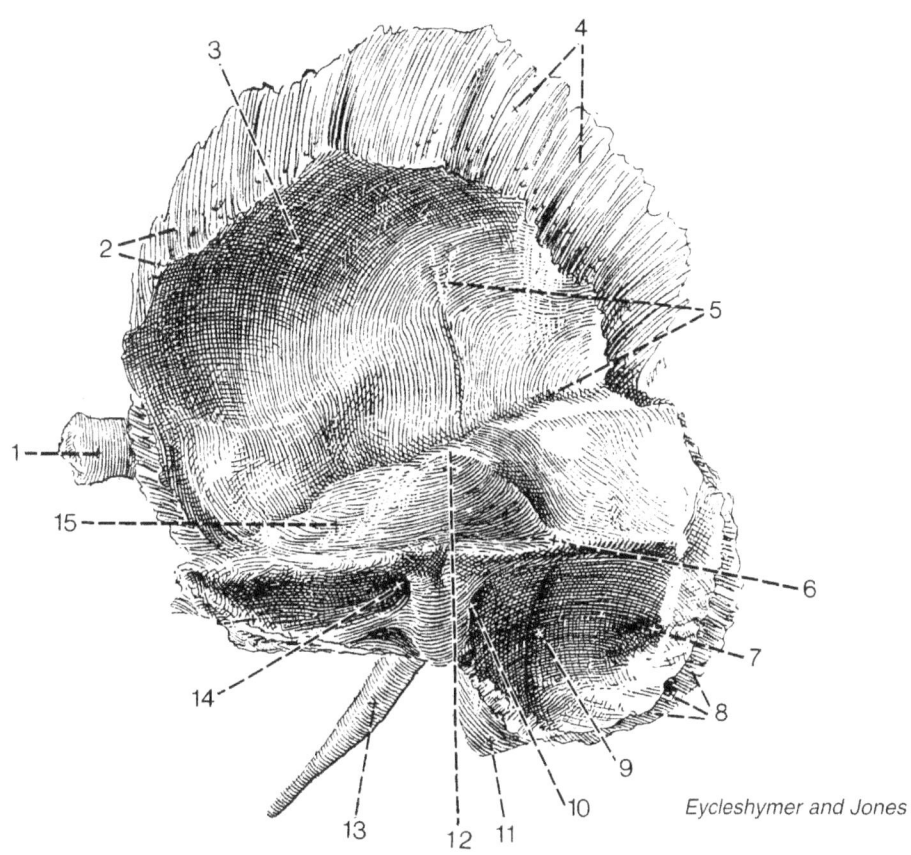

Eycleshymer and Jones

Color and label

1 Zygomatic process
2 Sphenoidal margin
3 Cerebral surface of squamous part
4 Parietal margin
5 Grooves for parietal branches of middle meningeal artery and accompanying veins
6 Groove for superior petrosal sinus
7 Mastoid foramen
8 Occipital margin
9 Sulcus for sigmoid sinus
10 Opening of vestibular aqueduct (contains endolymphatic duct, which forms endolymphatic sac at its end next to the dura mater)
11 Mastoid process
12 Arcuate eminence (marks position of anterior semicircular canal)
13 Styloid process
14 Internal acoustic opening (into which pass the facial nerve, vestibulocochlear nerve, and internal auditory artery)

1 _____
2 _____
3 _____
4 _____
5 _____
6 _____
7 _____
8 _____
9 _____
10 _____
11 _____
12 _____
13 _____
14 _____

H&N-25 Superficial muscles of the neck

The platysma has been removed.

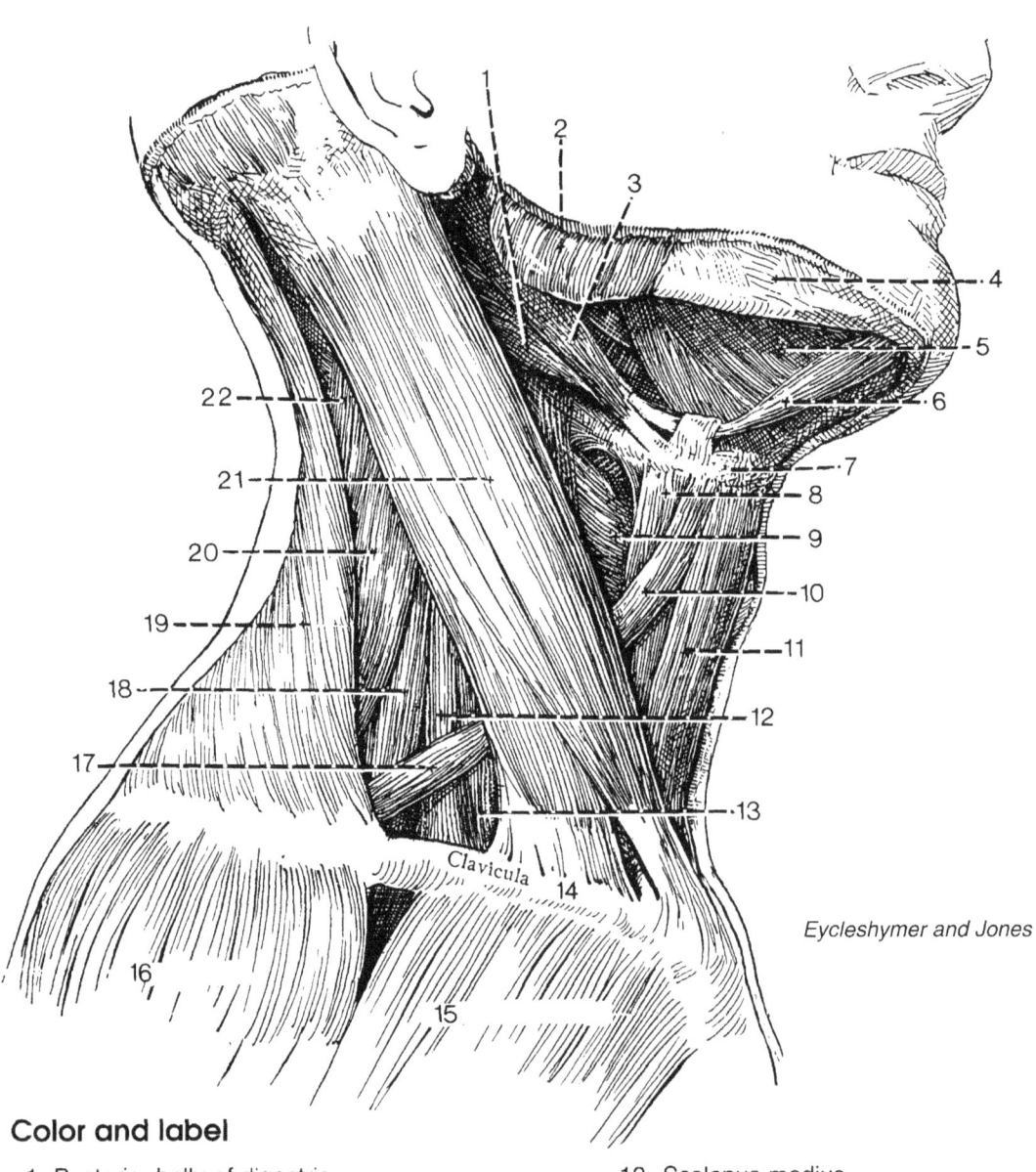

Eycleshymer and Jones

Color and label

1. Posterior belly of digastric
2. Masseter
3. Stylohyoid
4. Mandible
5. Mylohyoid
6. Anterior belly of digastric
7. Hyoid bone
8. Thyrohyoid
9. Inferior pharyngeal constrictor
10. Superior belly of omohyoid
11. Sternohyoid
12. Scalenus medius
13. Scalenus anterior
14. Clavicle
15. Pectoralis major
16. Deltoid
17. Inferior belly of omohyoid
18. Scalenus posterior
19. Trapezius
20. Levator scapulae
21. Sternocleidomastoid
22. Splenius capitis

H&N-25 Superficial muscles of the neck

The platysma has been removed.

(Opposite Page)

1 _____
2 _____
3 _____
4 _____
5 _____
6 _____
7 _____
8 _____
9 _____
10 _____
11 _____
12 _____
13 _____
14 _____
15 _____

16 _____
17 _____
18 _____
19 _____
20 _____
21 _____
22 _____

H&N-26 Left side of neck I

Platysma and deep cervical fascia have been removed

(opposite page)

Color and label

1. Body of mandible
2. Facial vein
3. Buccal fat pad
4. Facial artery
5. Marginal mandibular branch of facial nerve
6. Posterior belly of digastric muscle
7. Parotid gland
8. Posterior branch of retromandibular vein
9. Posterior auricular vein
10. Great auricular nerve
11. Lesser occipital nerve
12. Jugulodigastric lymph nodes
13. External jugular vein
14. Facial vein
15. Superior root of ansa cervicalis on internal carotid artery
16. Transverse cervical nerve (cut)
17. Accessory nerve (N XI) supplies trapezius and sternocleidomastoid muscles
18. Cervical nerves to trapezius
19. Trapezius muscle
20. Superficial cervical vein
21. Upper trunk of brachial plexus
22. Superficial cervical artery
23. Suprascapular nerve
24. Inferior belly of omohyoid muscle
25. Suprascapular artery
26. Scalenus anterior muscle
27. Supraclavicular nerves and their branches
28. Pectoralis major muscle
29. Phrenic nerve
30. Clavicular head of sternocleidomastoid muscle
31. Sternal head of sternocleidomastoid muscle
32. Inferior thyroid vein
33. Thyroid gland
34. Sternothyroid muscle
35. Superior belly of omohyoid muscle
36. Anterior jugular vein
37. Common carotid artery
38. Superior thyroid artery and external laryngeal nerve
39. Superior laryngeal artery
40. Internal laryngeal nerve
41. Nerve to thyrohyoid
42. Suprahyoid artery
43. Lingual artery
44. Body of hyoid bone
45. Hypoglossal nerve (N XII)
46. Anterior belly of digastric
47. Submandibular gland
48. Submental artery and vein
49. Sternohyoid muscle
50. Sternocleidomastoid muscle

1 _____
2 _____
3 _____
4 _____
5 _____
6 _____
7 _____
8 _____
9 _____
10 _____
11 _____
12 _____
13 _____
14 _____
15 _____
16 _____
17 _____
18 _____
19 _____
20 _____
21 _____
22 _____
23 _____
24 _____
25 _____

H&N-26 Left side of neck I

From the left and front

26 _____
27 _____
28 _____
29 _____
30 _____
31 _____
32 _____
33 _____
34 _____
35 _____
36 _____
37 _____
38 _____
39 _____
40 _____
41 _____
42 _____
43 _____
44 _____
45 _____
46 _____
47 _____
48 _____
49 _____
50 _____

Redrawn and slightly modified from McMinn and Hutchins

H&N-27 Left side of neck II

Deep dissection. Most of the sternocleidomastoid and submandibular gland have been removed.

Color and label (opposite page)

1. Hyoid bone
2. Anterior belly of digastric muscle
3. Suprahyoid artery
4. Marginal mandibular branch of facial nerve (N VII)
5. Submental artery
6. Facial artery
7. Vena comitans (Latin, vein running with) of hypoglossal nerve
8. Facial vein
9. Facial artery (arising from external carotid artery)
10. Hypoglossal nerve (N XII)
11. Stylohyoid muscle
12. Posterior belly of digastric muscle
13. Parotid gland
14. Sternocleidomastoid muscle (cut)
15. Second cervical nerve ventral ramus
16. Great auricular nerve
17. Carotid sinus at beginning of internal carotid artery (a baroreceptor or pressure receptor; the internal carotid gives off no branches in the neck)
18. Lesser occipital nerve
19. Third cervical nerve ventral ramus
20. Communicating ramus between nerves C3 and C4
21. Fourth cervical nerve ventral ramus
22. Fifth cervical nerve ventral ramus
23. Accessory nerve (N XI)
24. Scalenus medius muscle
25. Upper trunk of brachial plexus
26. Dorsal scapular nerve
27. Trapezius muscle (motor innervation: accessory nerve; sensory: cervical plexus)
28. Thyrohyoid muscle
29. Lingual artery
30. Internal laryngeal nerve
31. Superior laryngeal artery
32. External carotid artery
33. Superior thyroid artery
34. External laryngeal nerve
35. Common carotid artery
36. Internal jugular vein
37. Sternohyoid muscle
38. Superior belly of omohyoid
39. Sternothyroid muscle
40. Superior root of ansa cervicalis
41. Inferior root of ansa cervicalis
42. Ansa cervicalis (*ansa*, Latin, a loop or handle, probably related to a goose's neck, *anser*, goose)
43. Ramus of the ansa cervicalis to the infrahyoid muscles (also called strap muscles)
44. Omohyoid tendon
45. Inferior thyroid artery
46. Thyrocervical trunk (splitting into three arteries)
47. Clavicular head of sternocleidomastoid (cut)
48. Thoracic duct (emptying lymph into the subclavian vein)
49. Subclavian vein
50. Phrenic nerve (motor nerve to the diaphragm; arises mainly from cervical nerve C4)
51. Scalenus anterior muscle
52. Superficial cervical artery
53. Suprascapular artery
54. Suprascapular nerve
55. Inferior belly of omohyoid
56. Scalenus medius muscle

1 _____
2 _____
3 _____
4 _____
5 _____
6 _____
7 _____
8 _____
9 _____
10 _____
11 _____
12 _____
13 _____
14 _____
15 _____
16 _____
17 _____
18 _____
19 _____
20 _____
21 _____
22 _____
23 _____

H&N-27 Left side of neck II
Deep dissection

24 _____
25 _____
26 _____
27 _____
28 _____
29 _____
30 _____
31 _____
32 _____
33 _____
34 _____
35 _____
36 _____
37 _____
38 _____
39 _____
40 _____
41 _____
42 _____
43 _____
44 _____
45 _____
46 _____
47 _____
48 _____
49 _____
50 _____
51 _____
52 _____
53 _____
54 _____
55 _____
56 _____

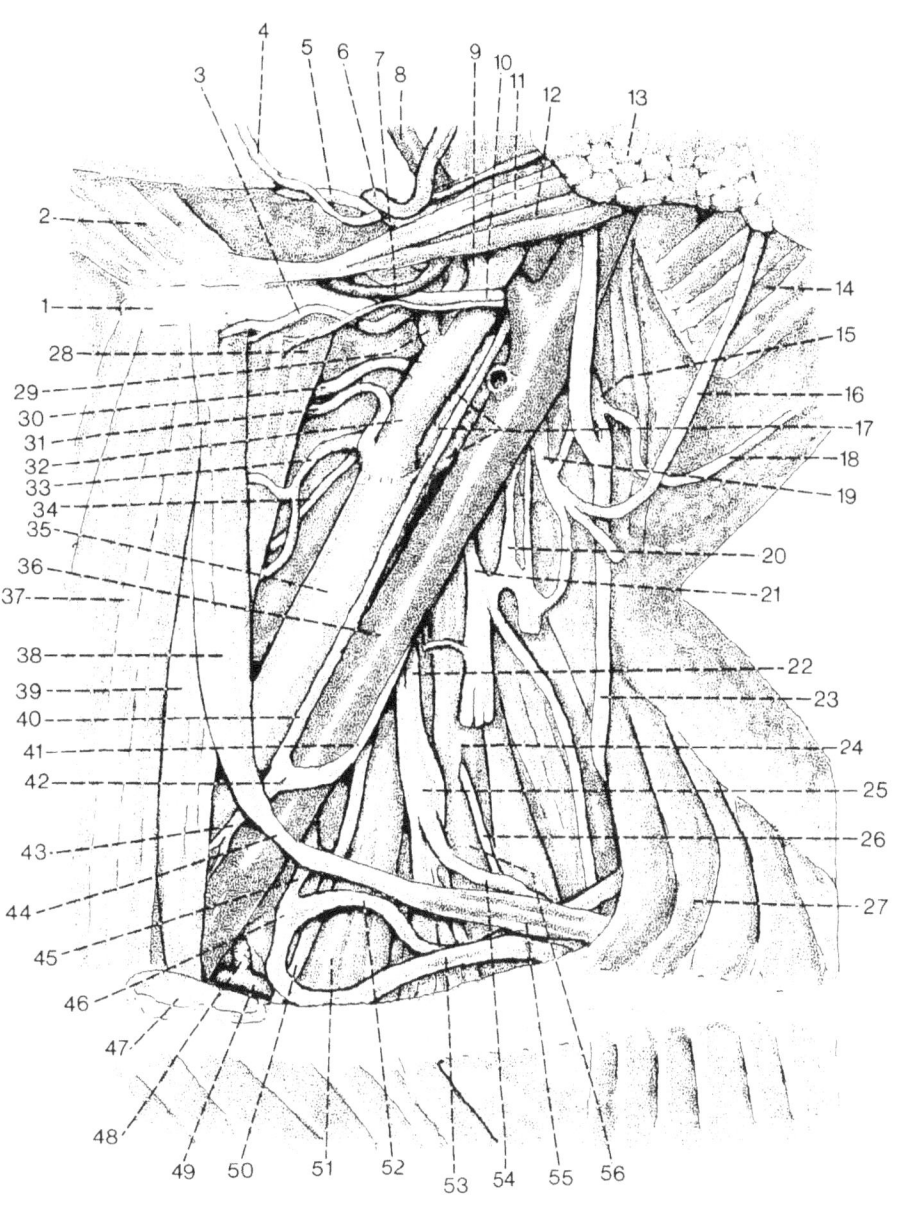

Redrawn from McMinn and Hutchins

H&N-28 Mandibular nerve and maxillary artery I

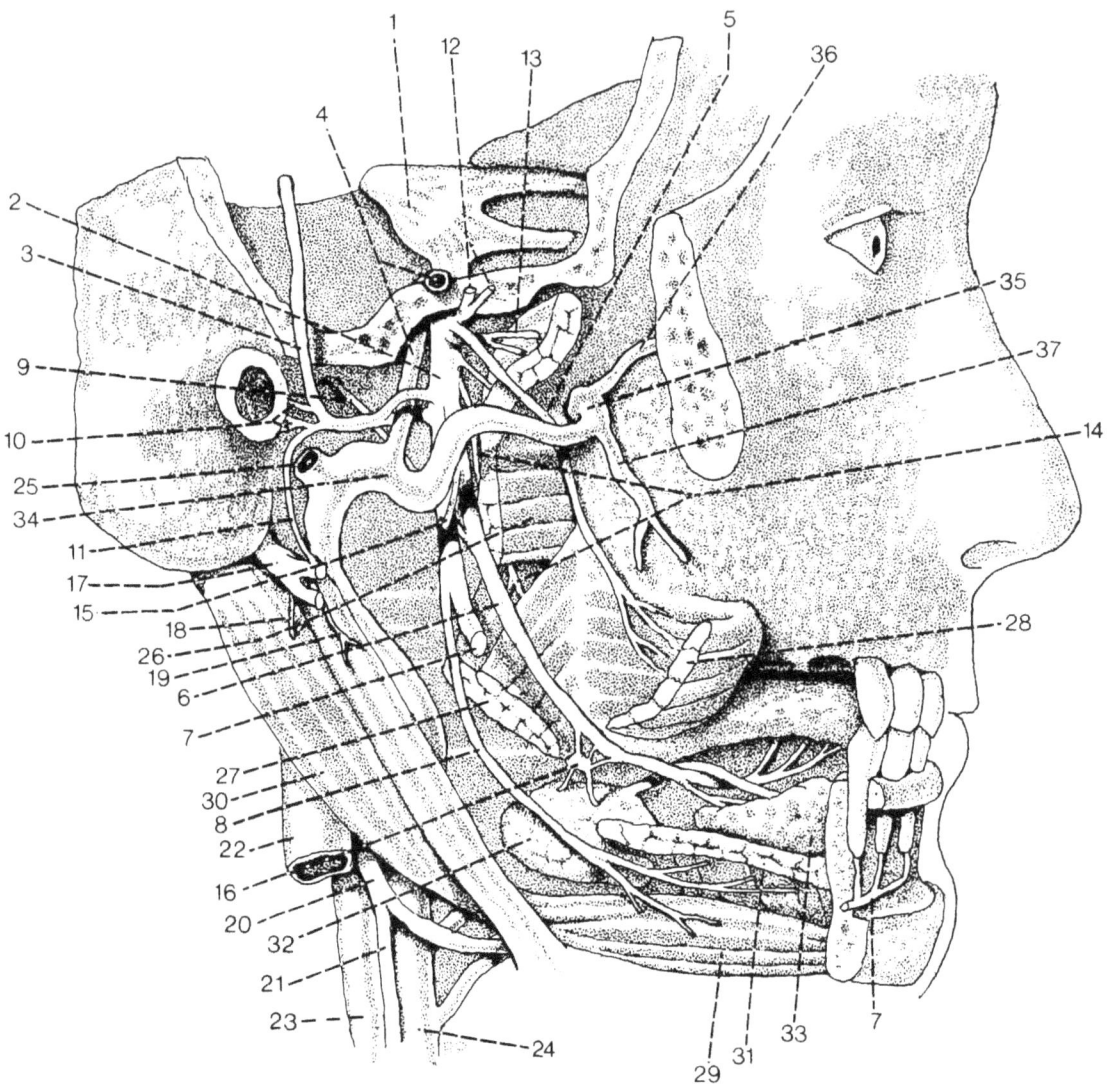

Color and label

1. Trigeminal ganglion
2. Mandibular nerve
3. Auriculotemporal nerve (notice its two roots surrounding the middle meningeal artery)
4. Middle meningeal artery
5. Buccal nerve (sensory to mucous membrane and skin of cheek)
6. Lingual nerve (supplies general sensation to anterior two-thirds of tongue)
7. Inferior alveolar nerve (cut)
8. Mylohyoid nerve (motor to mylohyoid muscle and anterior belly of digastric muscle)
9. Chorda tympani (branch of facial nerve carrying taste fibers and parasympathetic fibers to lingual nerve; exits skull through petrotympanic fissure)
10. External acoustic meatus nerves
11. Communicating branch with facial nerve
12. Deep temporal nerves (motor to temporalis muscle)
13. Lateral pterygoid nerve
14. Medial pterygoid nerve
15. Masseteric nerve
16. Submandibular ganglion
17. Facial nerve
18. Digastric branch of facial nerve (motor to posterior belly of digastric muscle)
19. Stylohyoid branch of facial nerve
20. Hypoglossal nerve
21. Superior root of ansa cervicalis
22. Internal jugular vein
23. Internal carotid artery
24. External carotid artery
25. Superficial temporal artery
26. Lateral pterygoid muscle (cut)
27. Medial pterygoid muscle (cut)
28. Buccinator muscle (cut and reflected)
29. Anterior belly of digastric muscle
30. Posterior belly of digastric muscle
31. Mylohyoid muscle (cut)
32. Sublingual gland (notice its duct crossing the lingual nerve)
33. Sublingual gland
34. Maxillary artery (most of its branches are not shown)
35. Sphenopalatine artery entering nasal cavity through sphenopalatine foramen
36. Infraorbital artery
37. Posterior superior alveolar artery

H&N-28 Mandibular nerve and maxillary artery I
(opposite page)

1. _____
2. _____
3. _____
4. _____
5. _____
6. _____
7. _____
8. _____
9. _____
10. _____
11. _____
12. _____
13. _____
14. _____
15. _____
16. _____
17. _____
18. _____
19. _____
20. _____

21. _____
22. _____
23. _____
24. _____
25. _____
26. _____
27. _____
28. _____
29. _____
30. _____
31. _____
32. _____
33. _____
34. _____
35. _____
36. _____
37. _____

H&N-29 Mandibular nerve and maxillary artery, II

Color and label

1. Right carotid artery
2. Maxillary artery
3. Superficial temporal artery (cut)
4. Middle meningeal artery (entering skull through foramen spinosum)
5. Posterior superior alveolar arteries
6. Infraorbital artery
7. Sphenopalatine artery
8. Pterygopalatine fossa
9. Sphenopalatine foramen
10. Mandibular nerve (exiting foramen ovale)
11. Deep temporal nerves (to temporal muscle)
12. Buccal nerve (sensory to cheek mucous membrane)
13. Lingual nerve (sensory to anterior two-thirds of tongue)
14. Inferior alveolar nerve (cut; sensory to teeth of lower jaw)
15. Mylohyoid nerve (to mylohyoid muscle and anterior belly of digastric)
16. Chorda tympani nerve (branch of facial nerve carrying taste from anterior two-thirds of tongue and parasympathetic fibers to sublingual and submandibular glands)
17. Auriculotemporal nerve (sensory to skin in front of ear and side of head)
18. Facial nerve (cut)
19. Posterior superior alveolar nerve (branch of maxillary nerve; sensory to upper posterior teeth)
20. Carotid canal
21. Jugular foramen
22. Styloid process (right and left)
23. Occipital condyle (right)
24. Hamulus of medial pterygoid plates (right and left)
25. Foramen magnum
26. Petrotympanic fissure
27. Stylomastoid foramen (facial nerve exits skull here)

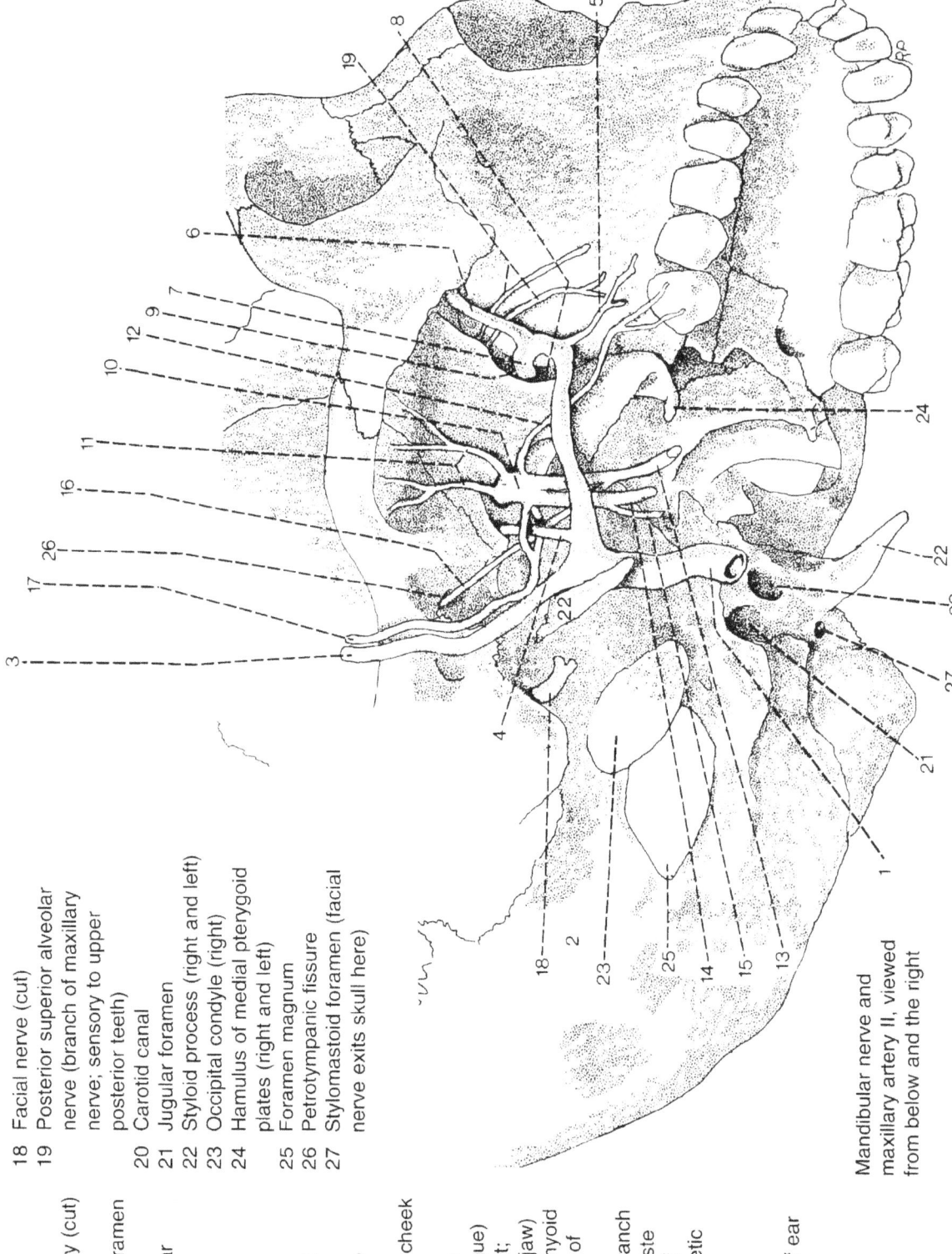

Mandibular nerve and maxillary artery II, viewed from below and the right

H&N-29 Mandibular nerve and maxillary artery, II (opposite page)

1. _____
2. _____
3. _____
4. _____
5. _____
6. _____
7. _____
8. _____
9. _____
10. _____
11. _____
12. _____
13. _____
14. _____
15. _____
16. _____
17. _____
18. _____
19. _____
20. _____
21. _____
22. _____
23. _____
24. _____
25. _____
26. _____
27. _____

H&N-30 The eyelid and eye in orbit

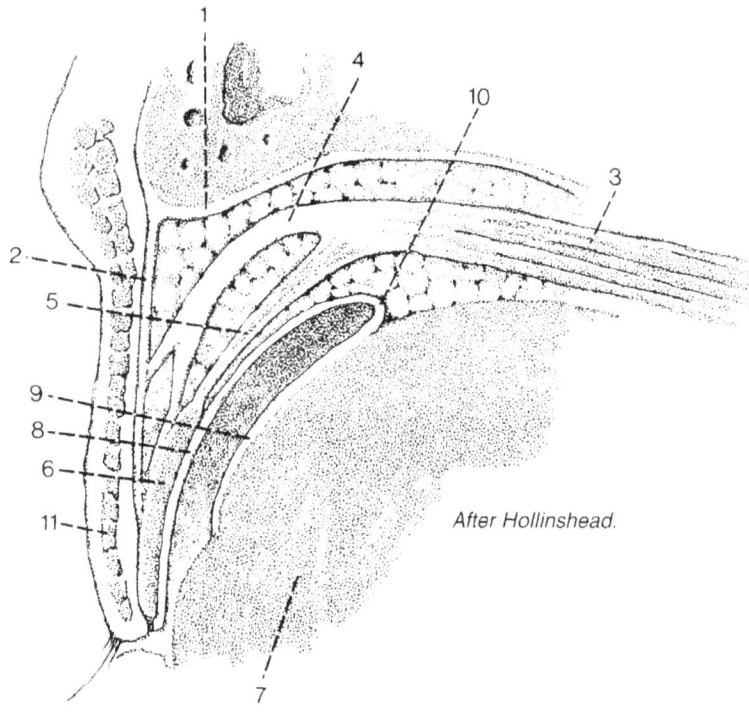

After Hollinshead.

Upper eyelid
Color and label

1. Periorbita (periosteum of the orbit)
2. Orbital septum (dense connective tissue sheet within eyelid, continuous with periorbita)
3. Levator palpebrae muscle (raiser of the upper lid)
4. Levator aponeurosis
5. Superior tarsal muscle (a smooth muscle supplied by sympathetic fibers)
6. Superior tarsus (a dense, curved plate of cartilage-like connective tissue)
7. Eyeball
8. Palpebral (eyelid) conjunctiva (a mucous membrane)
9. Bulbar (eyeball) conjunctiva (space between two layers of conjunctiva is exaggerated here; two layers slide against each other lubricated only by a thin layer of tears)
10. Superior conjunctival fornix (Latin, an arch)
11. Orbicularis oculi muscle (note muscle is within the upper lid as well as on the bony orbit)

Right eye and orbit
Color and label

1. Superior tarsus
2. Inferior tarsus
3. Tendon of levator palpebrae superior
4. Orbital septum
5. Lacrimal gland (orbital and palpebral parts)
6. Lateral palpebral ligament
7. Medial palpebral ligament (cut and relfected)
8. Superior lacrimal canaliculus
9. Inferior lacrimal canaliculus
10. Lacrimal sac
11. Nasolacrimal duct
12. Maxillary bone (cut open to show nasolacrimal duct)

After Wolf-Heidegger

H&N-30 The eyelid and eye in orbit (opposite page)

Upper eyelid
Color and label

1 _____
2 _____
3 _____
4 _____
5 _____
6 _____
7 _____
8 _____
9 _____
10 _____
11 _____

Right eye and orbit
Color and label

1 _____
2 _____
3 _____
4 _____
5 _____
6 _____
7 _____
8 _____
9 _____
10 _____
11 _____
12 _____

H&N-31 Extraocular muscles

Lateral view of right eye with lateral wall removed

Color and label

1 Superior rectus muscle
2 Lateral rectus muscle
3 Medial rectus muscle
4 Inferior rectus muscle
5 Superior oblique muscle
6 Inferior rectus muscle
7 Levator palpebrae muscle
 (also levator muscle of upper lid)
8 Anulus tendineus communis
 (also common tendinous ring)
9 Trochlea (Latin, pulley)
10 Optic nerve (cranial nerve II)
11 Bulbar conjunctiva (cut edge)
12 Frontal sinus
13 Maxillary sinus
14 Pterygopalatine fossa
15 Sphenopalatine foramen

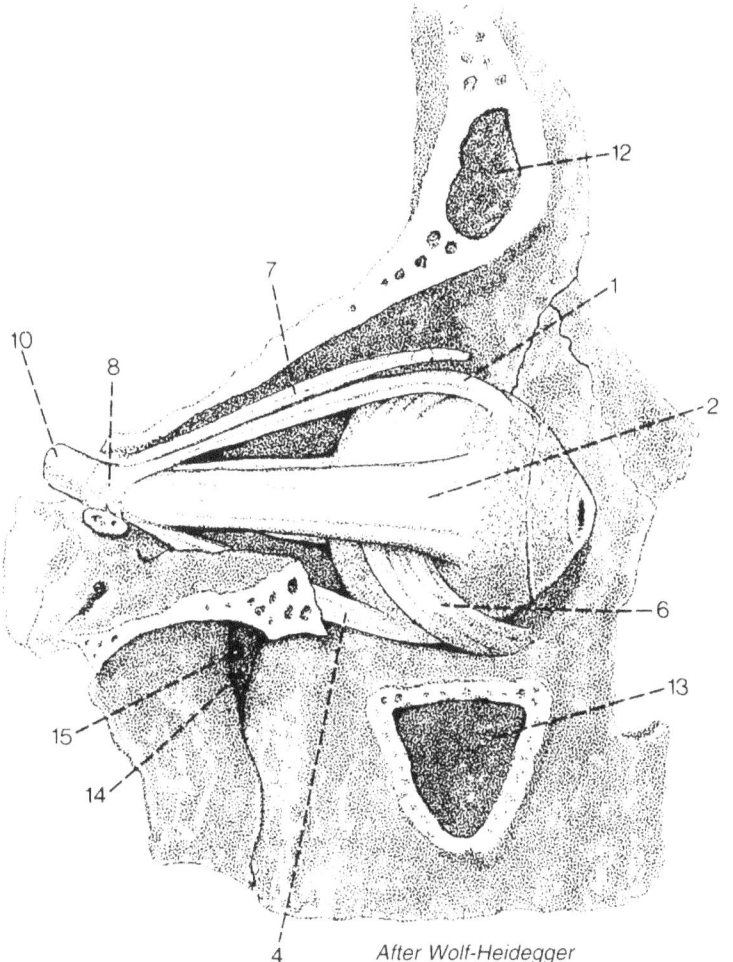

After Wolf-Heidegger

Superior view of right eye with roof of orbit removed

1 _____
2 _____
3 _____
4 _____
5 _____
6 _____
7 _____
8 _____
9 _____
10 _____
11 _____
12 _____
13 _____
14 _____
15 _____

H&N-32 Eye and orbit

Color and label (opposite page)

Figure A. Right eye

1. Pupil (central opening of iris, through which light enters)
2. Iris (pigmented; responsible for color of eye; blue, green, brown, etc.; regulates size of its central aperature, the pupil, by its circular sphincter muscle, which constricts the pupil, and its radial dilator muscle, which enlarges the pupil)
3. Reflection on cornea (the transparent cornea possesses a greater curvature than the eyeball itself; the curvature of the cornea is greatest in youth and least in old age; distortion of corneal curvature gives rise to astigmatism; more refraction of light occurs at the anterior surface of the cornea than in any other refractive media in the eye. In man the refractive power of the cornea is more than twice that of the lens)
4. Bulbar conjunctiva overlying sclera (sclera is white fibrous coat of eye)
5. Upper lid (palpebra superior)
6. Lower lid (palpebra inferior)
7. Cilia (eyelashes projecting from margin of eyelid)
8. Lacrimal caruncle (Latin, *lacrima*, a tear)

Figure B. Right orbit: anterior and slightly lateral view

1. Optic canal
2. Superior orbital fissure
3. Inferior orbital fissure
4. Infraorbital groove
5. Infraorbital canal and foramen
6. Fossa for lacrimal gland
7. Frontal bone
8. Zygomatic bone
9. Lacrimal bone
10. Probe in nasolacrimal duct
11. Orbital plate of ethmoid bone
12. Maxilla
13. Posterior lacrimal crest
14. Greater wing of sphenoid bone
15. Lesser wing of sphenoid bone
16. Nasal bone
17. Palatine bone

A (use abbrevs.)

1 _____
2 _____
3 _____
4 _____
5 _____
6 _____
7 _____
8 _____

B
1 _____   14 _____
2 _____   15 _____
3 _____   16 _____
4 _____   17 _____
5 _____
6 _____
7 _____
8 _____
9 _____
10 _____
11 _____
12 _____
13 _____

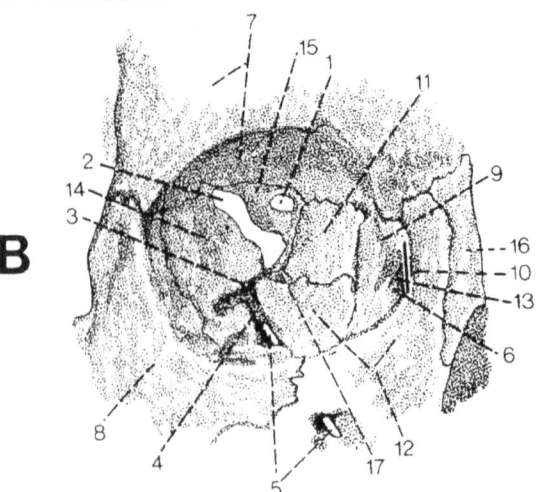

50

H&N-32 Eye and orbit

Anterior aspect

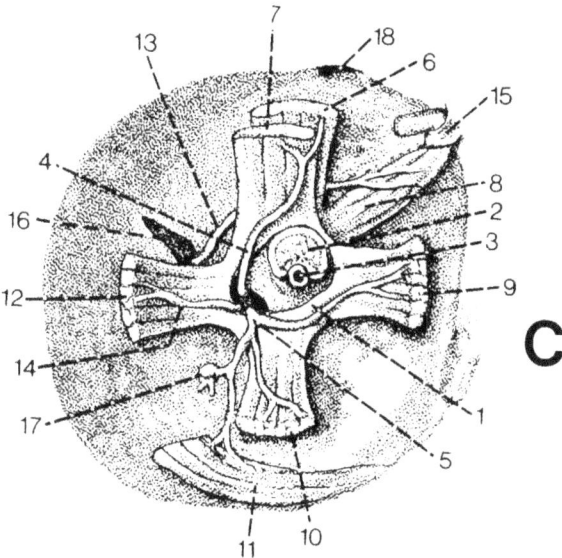

Figure C. Common tendinous ring (anulus tendineus communis)

1. Common tendinous ring (notice that it encircles the optic canal, including the optic nerve and ophthalmic artery, and also encircles part of the superior orbital fissure with the abducent nerve and oculomotor nerve)
2. Optic nerve emerging from the optic canal
3. Ophthalmic artery
4. Superior ramus of oculomotor nerve (innervates superior rectus and levator palpebrae muscles)
5. Inferior ramus of oculomotor nerve (innervates medial rectus, inferior rectus, and inferior oblique muscles)
6. Levator palpebrae muscle
7. Superior rectus muscle
8. Superior oblique muscle
9. Medial rectus muscle
10. Inferior rectus muscle
11. Inferior oblique muscle
12. Lateral rectus muscle
13. Trochlear nerve
14. Abducent nerve
15. Trochlea (Latin, a pulley)
16. Superior orbital fissure
17. Ciliary ganglion (contains postganglionic parasympathetic nerve cell bodies that cause constriction of the pupil and greater curvature of the lens for near vision)
18. Supraorbital notch

1 _____
2 _____
3 _____
4 _____
5 _____
6 _____
7 _____
8 _____
9 _____

10 _____
11 _____
12 _____
13 _____
14 _____
15 _____
16 _____
17 _____
18 _____

H&N-33 Nerves of the orbit
Superior aspect

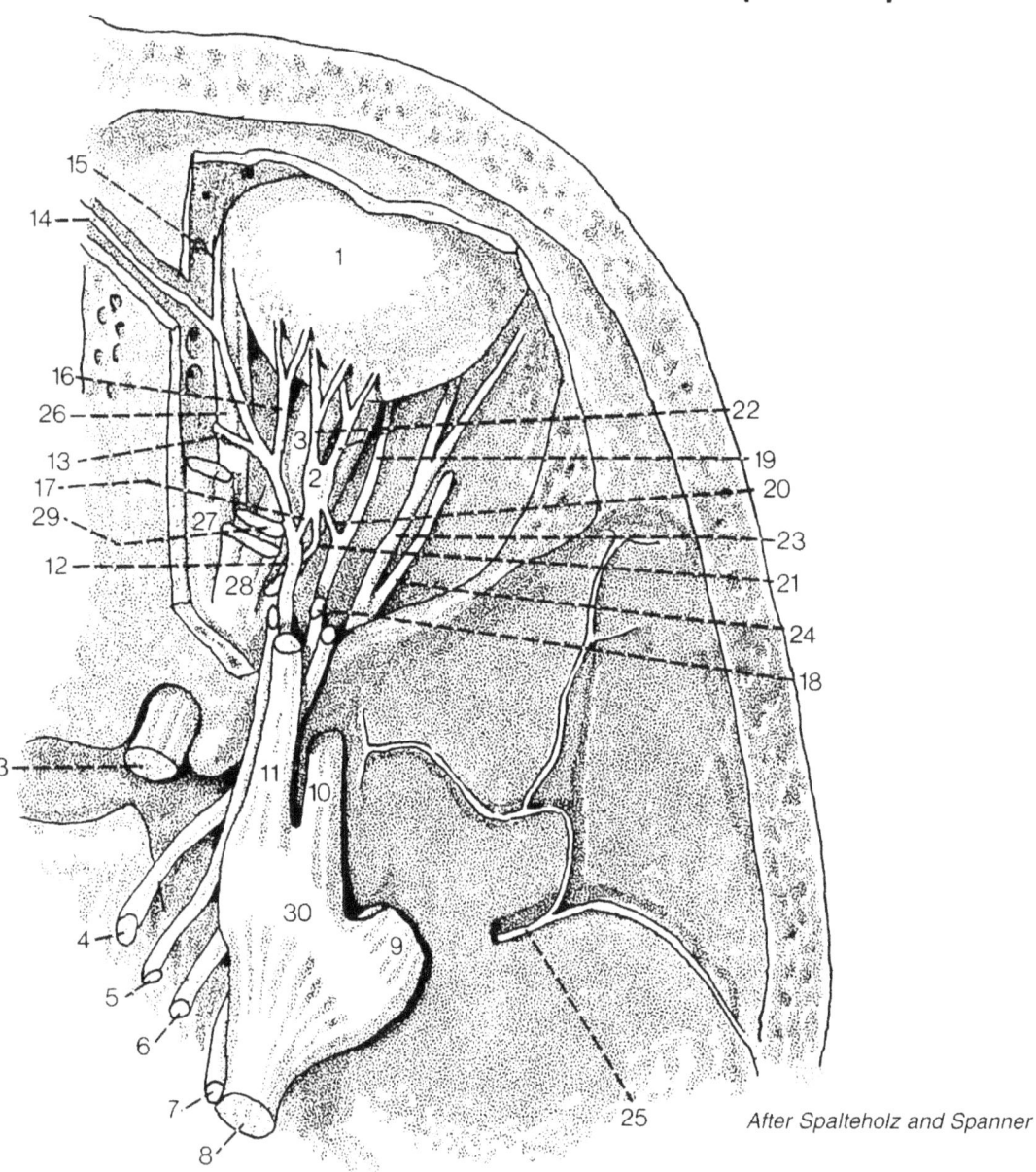

After Spalteholz and Spanner

Color and label

1. Eyeball
2. Ciliary ganglion (parasympathetic)
3. Optic nerve (II)
4. Oculomotor nerve (III)
5. Trochlear nerve (IV)
6. Abducent nerve (VI)
7. Motor root (portio minor) of trigeminal nerve (V)
8. Sensory root (portio major) of trigeminal nerve (V)
9. Mandibular nerve (major branch of trigeminal nerve)
10. Maxillary nerve (major branch of trigeminal nerve)
11. Ophthalmic nerve (major branch of trigeminal nerve; cut)
12. Nasociliary nerve (branch of ophthalmic nerve)
13. Posterior ethmoidal nerve
14. Anterior ethmoidal nerve
15. Infratrochlear
16. Long ciliary nerves
17. Communicating branch of nasociliary nerve with ciliary ganglion
18. Oculomotor nerve superior branch (cut)
19. Oculomotor nerve inferior branch
20. Oculomotor root of ciliary ganglion
21. Sympathetic branch to ciliary ganglion
22. Short ciliary nerves
23. Zygomatic nerve
24. Infraorbital nerve
25. Meningeal branch of mandibular nerve
26. Medial rectus muscle
27. Superior oblique muscle (cut)
28. Levator palpebrae superior muscle (cut)
29. Superior rectus muscle (cut)
30. Trigeminal ganglion

H&N-33 Nerves of the orbit
Superior aspect
(opposite page)

1 _____

2 _____

3 _____

4 _____

5 _____

6 _____

7 _____

8 _____

9 _____

10 _____

11 _____

12 _____

13 _____

14 _____

15 _____

16 _____

17 _____

18 _____

19 _____

20 _____

21 _____

22 _____

23 _____

24 _____

25 _____

26 _____

27 _____

28 _____

29 _____

30 _____

H&N-34 Nerves of the orbit
Lateral aspect

The bones of the right orbit and part of the right maxilla are removed, showing roots of the teeth and their innervation.

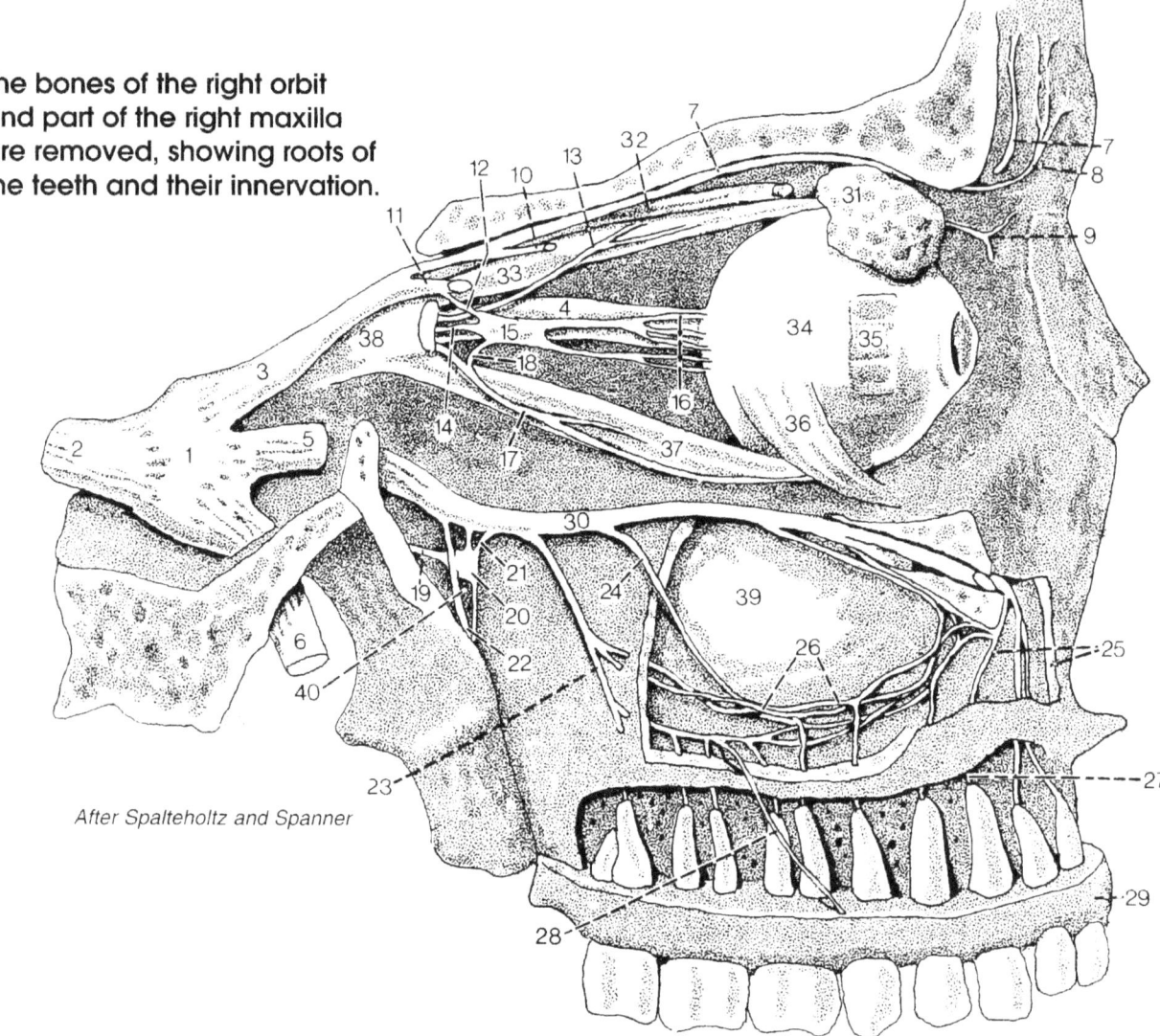

After Spalteholtz and Spanner

Color and label

1. Trigeminal (semilunar) ganglion
2. Sensory root of trigeminal nerve
3. Ophthalmic nerve (V_1)
4. Optic nerve
5. Maxillary nerve (V_2)
6. Mandibular nerve (V_3) (cut)
7. Supraorbital nerve
8. Supraorbital nerve (medial branch)
9. Supratrochlear nerve
10. Lacrimal nerve (cut)
11. Nasociliary nerve (cut)
12. Branch from nasociliary nerve to ciliary ganglion
13. Superior branch of oculomotor nerve
14. Sympathetic branch to ciliary ganglion
15. Ciliary ganglion
16. Short ciliary nerves
17. Inferior branch of oculomotor nerve
18. Oculomotor root to ciliary ganglion
19. Nerve of pterygoid canal
20. Pterygopalatine ganglion
21. Pterygopalatine nerves
22. Palatine nerves
23. Posterior superior alveolar branches
24. Middle superior alveolar branches
25. Anterior superior alveolar branches
26. Superior dental plexus
27. Superior dental branches
28. Gingival branch
29. Gingiva (Latin, *gingiva*, the gum)
30. Infraorbital nerve
31. Lacrimal gland
32. Levator palpebrae superior muscle
33. Superior rectus muscle
34. Eyeball
35. Lateral rectus muscle (cut)
36. Inferior oblique muscle
37. Inferior rectus muscle
38. Common tendinous ring
39. Mucous membrane of maxillary sinus
40. Pterygopalatine fossa

H&N-34 Nerves of the orbit

Lateral aspect

(opposite page)

1 _____
2 _____
3 _____
4 _____
5 _____
6 _____
7 _____
8 _____
9 _____
10 _____
11 _____
12 _____
13 _____
14 _____
15 _____
16 _____
17 _____
18 _____
19 _____
20 _____
21 _____
22 _____
23 _____
24 _____
25 _____
26 _____
27 _____
28 _____
29 _____
30 _____
31 _____
32 _____
33 _____
34 _____
35 _____
36 _____
37 _____
38 _____
39 _____
40 _____

H&N-35 Lower half of right eye

Upper figure is an enlarged segment of the area marked by dashed lines in the lower figure.

(opposite page)

Color and label

1. Cornea (the anterior, transparent, curved portion of the outer fibrous tunic of the eyeball)
2. Iris (the colored, visible portion of the middle vascular tunic of the eye; functions as a diaphragm with the central opening, the pupil, capable of enlarging or contracting, thus controlling the amount of light entering the eye)
3. Anterior chamber (lies behind the cornea and in front of the iris and the central part of the lens; filled with aqueous humor)
4. Posterior chamber (a narrow circular space behind the iris and in front of the peripheral part of the lens and the anterior zonule fibers; also filled with aqueous humor)
5. Lens. The biconvex lens is held in place by the surrounding zonule fibers, which are attached to its periphery. The natural tendency of the lens is to assume a more curved or globular shape; this allows it to focus light from near objects. Apposed to this is the radial outward pull of the zonule fibers, which extend from the surrounding ciliary processes to the lens; their outward pull causes the lens to become flatter and allow the lens to focus light from far objects. The shape of the lens depends upon the surrounding circular ciliary muscles. Contraction of the circular ciliary muscles reduces the diameter of the ciliary body and thereby lessens the outward pull on the edge of the lens, thus allowing the lens to become more biconvex and focus on near objects; this is accommodation. Presbyopia, or "old vision," is the loss of ability to focus on close objects, as in reading, due to the thickening of the lens, which occurs with advanced age, resulting in the loss of lens elasticity and an inability of the lens to assume the more curved biconvex form.
6. Ciliary processes (these are about 70 tiny radially-arranged, wrinkled folds; they lie in the pars plica or folded part of the ciliary body; also called ciliary crown)
7. Ciliary body (muscular part); this completely encircles the lens and consists of smooth muscle that controls the curvature of the lens; the muscles of accommodation
8. Anterior zonule fibers (these attach to the front of the lens where they fuse with the lens capsule)
9. Posterior zonule fibers (these attach to the back of the lens where they fuse with the lens capule)
10. Trabecular meshwork (this is an irregular network of tiny beams or trabeculae at the periphery of the anterior chamber where the iris joins the cornea; the convoluted passages between the trabeclae contain aqueous humor which slowly flows outward eventually to be absorbed by the scleral venous sinus or canal of Schlemm)
11. Scleral venous sinus or canal of Schlemm (this vein encircles the inner part of the corneoscleral junction; it drains the aqueous humor from the anterior chamber of the eye; **glaucoma** is an increase in intraocular pressure sufficient to damage the function or structure of the eye; caused by the blockage of drainage and buildup of aqueous humor in the anterior chamber; *glaukoma*, Greek, gleaming, bluish green, gray)
12. Limbus (the corneoscleral junction)
13. Conjunctiva (bulbar conjunctiva is the transparent mucous membrane on the sclera; it is also reflected onto the inner surface of both upper and lower lids as palpebral conjunctiva)
14. Sclera (the white, fibrous, outer coat of the eyeball)
15. Choroid (the middle, vascular tunic of the eyeball)
16. Retina (the inner, nervous, light-sensitive tunic of the eye)
17. Fovea centralis (the central part of the retina responsible for maximum visual acuity; contains only tightly-packed cones)
18. Outer dural sheath of optic nerve
19. Central artery and vein of the retina
20. Optic nerve
21. Ciliary body (pars plana or smooth part; covered by the non-nervous part of the retina)

H&N-35 Lower half of right eye
(opposite page)

(use abbrevs.)

1 _____
2 _____
3 _____
4 _____
5 _____
6 _____
7 _____
8 _____
9 _____
10 _____
11 _____
12 _____
13 _____
14 _____
15 _____
16 _____
17 _____
18 _____
19 _____
20 _____
21 _____

H&N-36 Principal veins of face and orbit

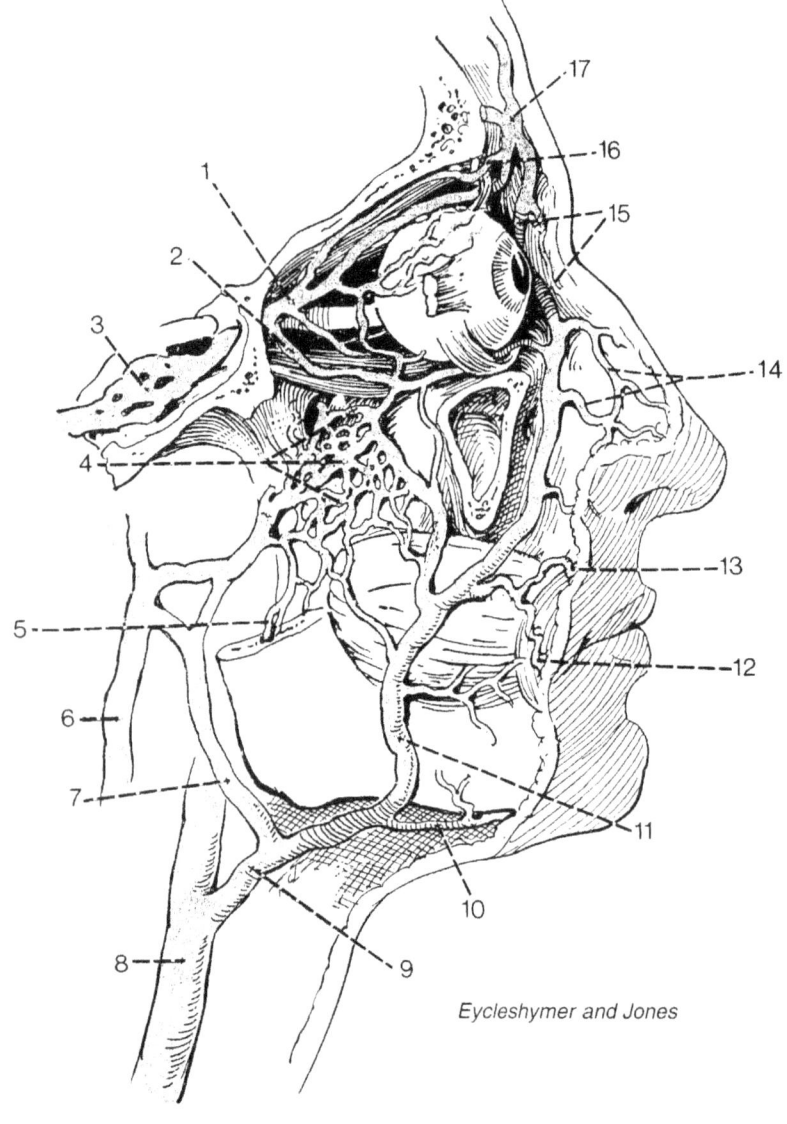

Eycleshymer and Jones

1 _____
2 _____
3 _____
4 _____
5 _____
6 _____
7 _____
8 _____
9 _____
10 _____
11 _____
12 _____
13 _____
14 _____
15 _____
16 _____
17 _____

Color and label

1 Superior ophthalmic vein
2 Inferior ophthalmic vein
3 Cavernous sinus
4 Pterygoid plexus
5 Inferior alveolar vein (doubled)
6 External jugular vein
7 Retromandibular vein
8 Internal jugular vein
9 Facial vein
10 Submental vein
11 Facial vein
12 Inferior labial vein
13 Superior labial vein
14 External nasal veins
15 Angular vein
16 Supraorbital vein
17 Anastomosis of angular vein with supraorbital and supratrochlear veins

H&N-37 The lacrimal apparatus

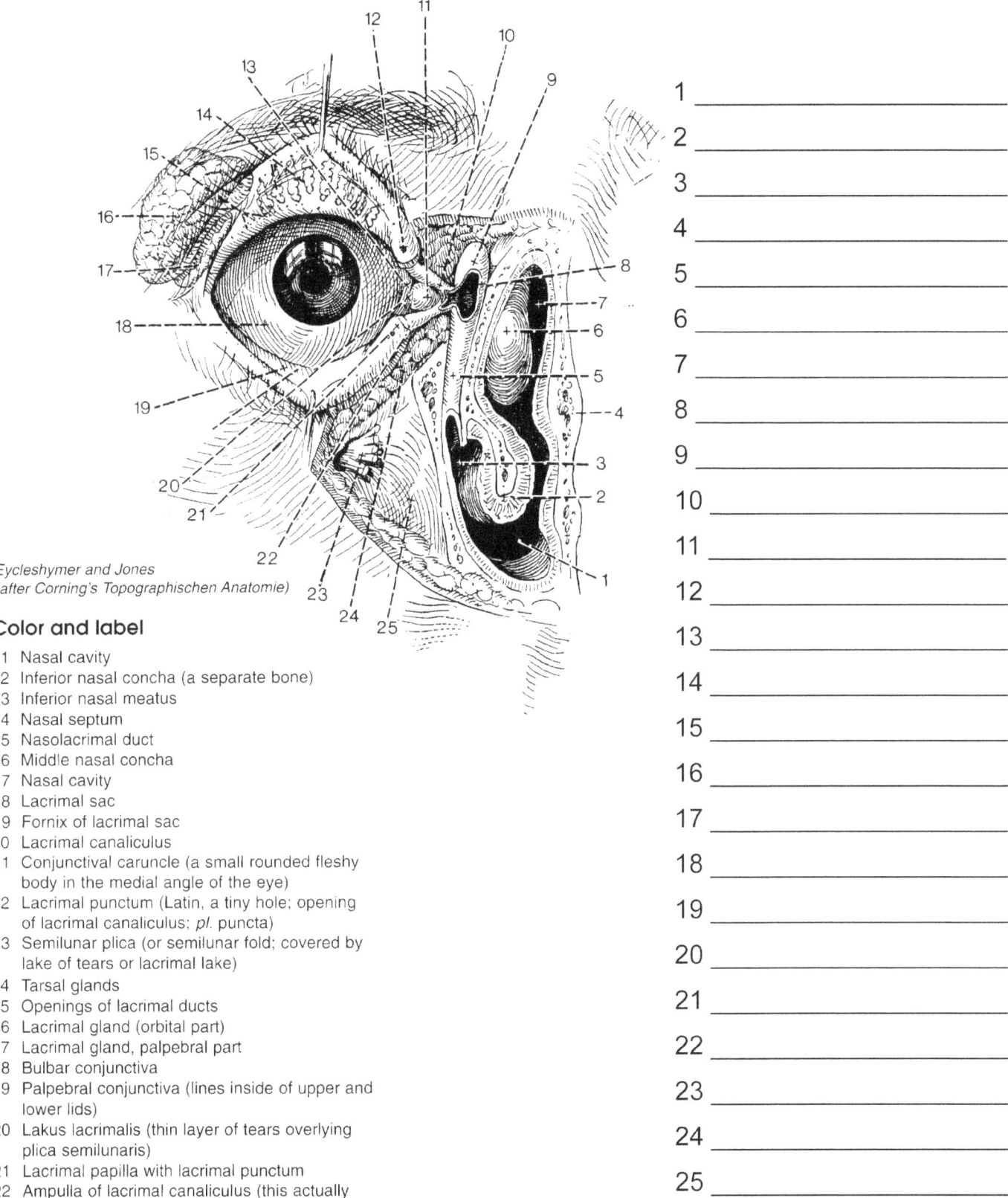

Eycleshymer and Jones
(after Corning's Topographischen Anatomie)

Color and label

1. Nasal cavity
2. Inferior nasal concha (a separate bone)
3. Inferior nasal meatus
4. Nasal septum
5. Nasolacrimal duct
6. Middle nasal concha
7. Nasal cavity
8. Lacrimal sac
9. Fornix of lacrimal sac
10. Lacrimal canaliculus
11. Conjunctival caruncle (a small rounded fleshy body in the medial angle of the eye)
12. Lacrimal punctum (Latin, a tiny hole; opening of lacrimal canaliculus; *pl.* puncta)
13. Semilunar plica (or semilunar fold; covered by lake of tears or lacrimal lake)
14. Tarsal glands
15. Openings of lacrimal ducts
16. Lacrimal gland (orbital part)
17. Lacrimal gland, palpebral part
18. Bulbar conjunctiva
19. Palpebral conjunctiva (lines inside of upper and lower lids)
20. Lakus lacrimalis (thin layer of tears overlying plica semilunaris)
21. Lacrimal papilla with lacrimal punctum
22. Ampulla of lacrimal canaliculus (this actually occurs at the "elbow" or bend in the lacrimal canaliculus)
23. Infraorbital nerve
24. Orbital fat
25. Maxilla

H&N-38 Dissection of ear and cast of bony labyrinth
(opposite page)

Color and label
Figure A
1. Pinna (also called auricle)
2. Cartilaginous walls of external acoustic (or auditory) meatus; walls are cartilage externally and bone internally
3. External acoustic meatus; contains ceruminous glands that produce the orange-brown ear wax, or cerumen, which, when accumulated in excess amounts, may impair hearing
4. Bony wall of external auditory meatus; this canal is about 2.5 cm long and acts as a resonator for sound waves in the critical range of human speech (2000 to 4000 cycles per second), thus amplifying these sounds.
5. Umbo of the ear drum; the ear drum (or tympanic membrane) is shaped like a blunt cone, with the deepest point externally called the umbo (Latin for the raised ornament on a shield); the outside of the ear drum is skin and is supplied by sensory fibers from nerves V and X; because the vagus nerve (X) also supplies the pharynx and larynx, an object lodged against the ear drum may produce a cough.
6. Middle ear cavity; lined with a mucous membrane that covers the walls, the 3 ossicles, their ligaments, and nerves; under certain conditions mucus may accumulate in the middle ear to the point that the normal vibratory movements of the ear drum and 3 ear ossicles are impeded and hearing is impaired; **otitis media** is a general term for inflammation of the middle ear; cranial nerve IX supplies sensory fibers to the middle ear and inner surface of the ear drum; the middle ear is filled with air and communicates with the nasopharynx by way of the auditory tune.
7. Internal jugular vein (note its proximity to the middle ear)
8. Round window (fenestra cochleae); closed by a membrane that acts as a pressure release for waves in the perilymph in the cochlea; it bulges out when the foot plate of the stapes pushes in at the oval window.
9. Vestibule; the fluid-filled cavity within the temporal bone containing the membranous utricle and the saccule.
10. Auditory tube; old name, eustachian tube; this connects the middle ear with the nasopharynx; normally closed, when dilated, as in yawning, it allows air in the middle ear to equalize with the ambient air pressure.
11. Nasopharynx
12. Malleus (Latin, hammer); note that the end of the malleus handle is attached to the inside of the ear drum at the umbo.
13. Incus (Latin, anvil)
14. Lateral semicircular canal; each semicircular canal contains a thinner semicircular duct.
15. Posterior semicircular canal
16. Anterior semicircular canal
17. Facial nerve (N VII; cut)
18. Internal acoustic meatus
19. Vestibulocochlear nerve (VIII)
20. Cochlea (Latin, a snail); the snail-like tubular spiral divided into 3 scalae or compartments: (1) the tympani, (2) the scala media or cochlea duct, and (3) the scala vestibuli.
21. Footplate (or base) of stapes (Latin, stirrup); it covers the oval window; sound-induced vibrations of the footplate send pressure waves into the endolymph of the vestibule which are simultaneously carried into the cochlea.

H&N-38 Dissection of ear and cast of bony labyrinth

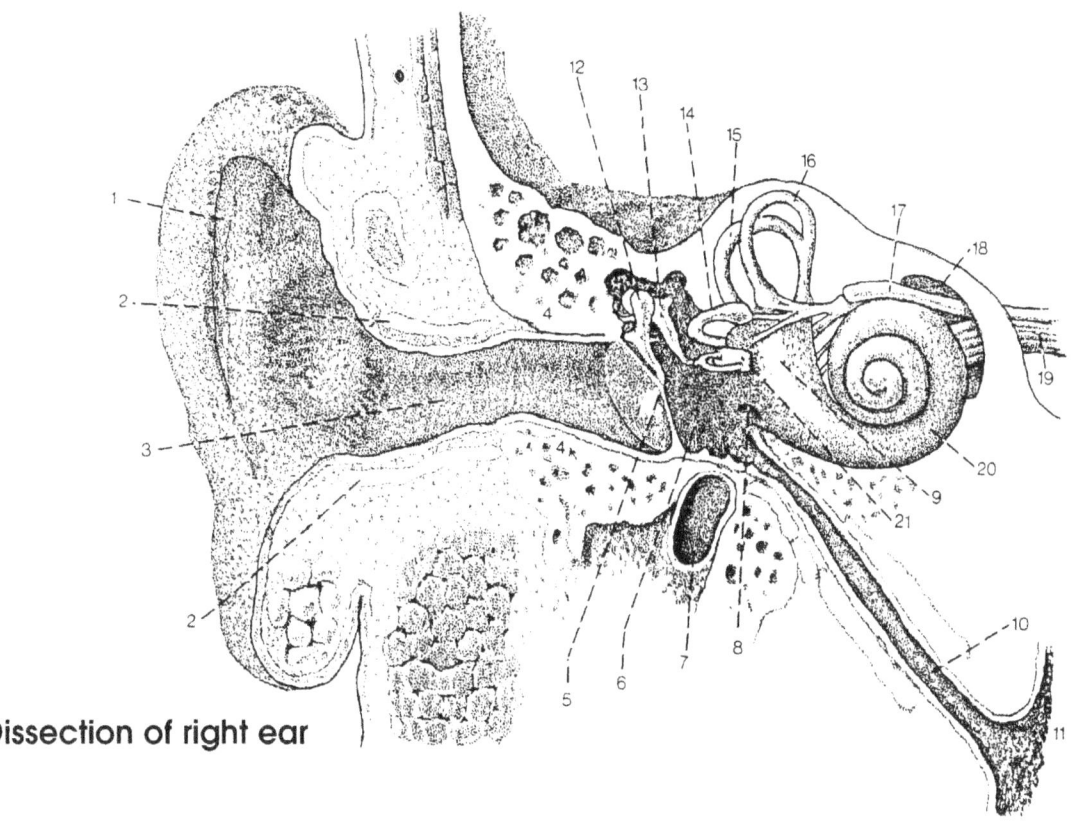

Figure A. Dissection of right ear

(use abbrevs.)

1 _____
2 _____
3 _____
4 _____
5 _____
6 _____
7 _____
8 _____
9 _____
10 _____
11 _____

12 _____
13 _____
14 _____
15 _____
16 _____
17 _____
18 _____
19 _____
20 _____
21 _____

H&N-38 Dissection of ear and cast of bony labyrinth

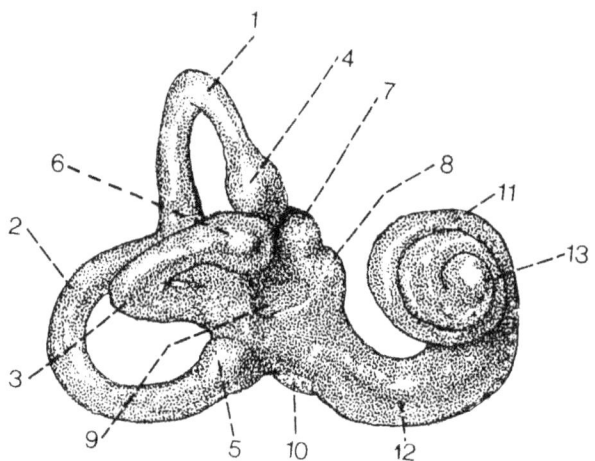

Figure B. Bony labyrinth

Right bony labyrinth (from a cast)

Color and label

1. Anterior semicircular canal
2. Posterior semicircular canal
3. Lateral semicircular canal
4. Anterior bony ampulla
5. Posterior bony ampulla
6. Lateral bony ampulla
7. Elliptical recess
8. Spherical recess
9. Fenestra vestibuli (former name: oval window)
10. Fenestra cochleae (former name: round window)
11. Cochlea
12. Base of cochlea
13. Cupula of cochlea

Based on Spalteholz and Spanner

Figure B
The bony labyrinth is a series of cavities and canals within the petrous portion of the temporal bone. The thinner membranous labyrinth lies within the bony labyrinth. The membranous labyrinth contains endolymph. The outer bony labyrinth contains perilymph, which surrounds and bathes the membranous labyrinth.

1 _____
2 _____
3 _____
4 _____
5 _____
6 _____
7 _____
8 _____
9 _____
10 _____
11 _____
12 _____
13 _____

H&N-39 Dissection of ear

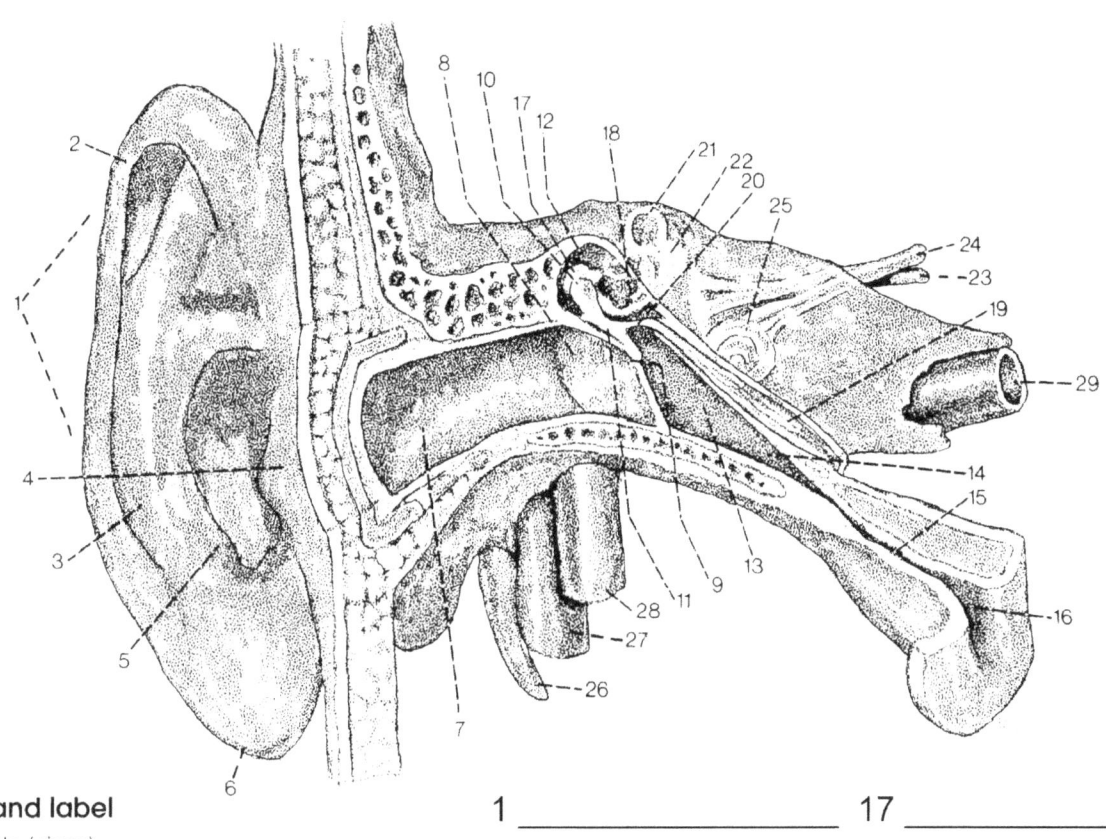

Color and label

1. Auricle (pinna)
2. Helix
3. Antihelix
4. Tragus
5. Antitragus
6. Lobule of auricle
7. External acoustic meatus
8. Tympanic membrane (eardrum)
9. Umbo of tympanic membrane
10. Head of malleus
11. Handle of malleus (attached at umbo)
12. Epitympanic recess
13. Middle ear (tympanic cavity)
14. Auditory tube (bony part)
15. Auditory tube (cartilaginous part)
16. Pharyngeal opening of auditory tube in nasal pharynx
17. Incus
18. Stapes
19. Tensor tympani muscle
20. Tendon of tensor tympani inserting on malleus
21. Superior semicircular canal (within petrous part of temporal bone)
22. Vestibule (cavity containing both utricle and saccule)
23. Vestibular nerve (of vestibulocochlear nerve)
24. Cochlear nerve (of vestibulocochlear nerve)
25. Cochlea
26. Styloid process
27. Internal jugular vein
28. Internal carotid artery (entering carotid canal)
29. Internal carotid artery (emerging from carotid canal)

H&N-40 Middle ear and ear ossicles

(opposite page)

Color and label
Figure A. Right middle ear, anterior view

1. External acoustic meatus
2. Tympanic membrane (ear drum; cut in half)
3. Umbo (central deepest point on exterior of tympanic membrane)
4. Fibrocartilaginous ring
5. Tympanic cavity (middle ear cavity, auris media)
6. Handle of malleus
7. Head of malleus
8. Body of incus
9. Long leg of incus
10. Head of stapes
11. Anterior leg of stapes
12. Posterior leg of stapes
13. Base (footplate) of stapes; covering oval window (fenestra vestibuli)
14. Perilymph in inner ear
15. Facial nerve in canal (cut)
16. Lateral mallear ligament
17. Lateral mallear process
18. Insertion of tensor tympani tendon (cut) on handle of malleus
19. Superior mallear ligament
20. Superior incudial ligament

1 _____   13 _____
2 _____   14 _____
3 _____   15 _____
4 _____   16 _____
5 _____   17 _____
6 _____   18 _____
7 _____   19 _____
8 _____   20 _____
9 _____
10 _____
11 _____
12 _____

Figures B and C. Right middle ear viewed from the inside looking out. Stapes has been removed.

Color and label

1. Tympanic membrane
2. Handle of malleus (attached to inside of ear drum at umbo)
3. Insertion of tensor tympani tendon on handle of malleus
4. Chorda tympani nerve (a branch of facial nerve)
5. Head of malleus
6. Body of incus
7. Short leg of incus
8. Long leg of incus
9. Lenticular process of incus (shaped like a small lentil bean)
10. Auditory tube (formerly, eustachian tube)
11. Canal for tensor tympani muscle (muscle has been removed)
12. Superior mallear ligament
13. Superior incudial ligament
14. Posterior incudial ligament
15. Anterior mallear fold
16. Posterior mallear fold
17. Fibrocartilaginous ring of tympanic membrane
18. Facial nerve
19. Anterior tympanic recess
20. Posterior tympanic recess

1 _____   13 _____
2 _____   14 _____
3 _____   15 _____
4 _____   16 _____
5 _____   17 _____
6 _____   18 _____
7 _____   19 _____
8 _____   20 _____
9 _____
10 _____
11 _____
12 _____

H&N-40 Middle ear and ear ossicles

Tympanic membrane and ear ossicles

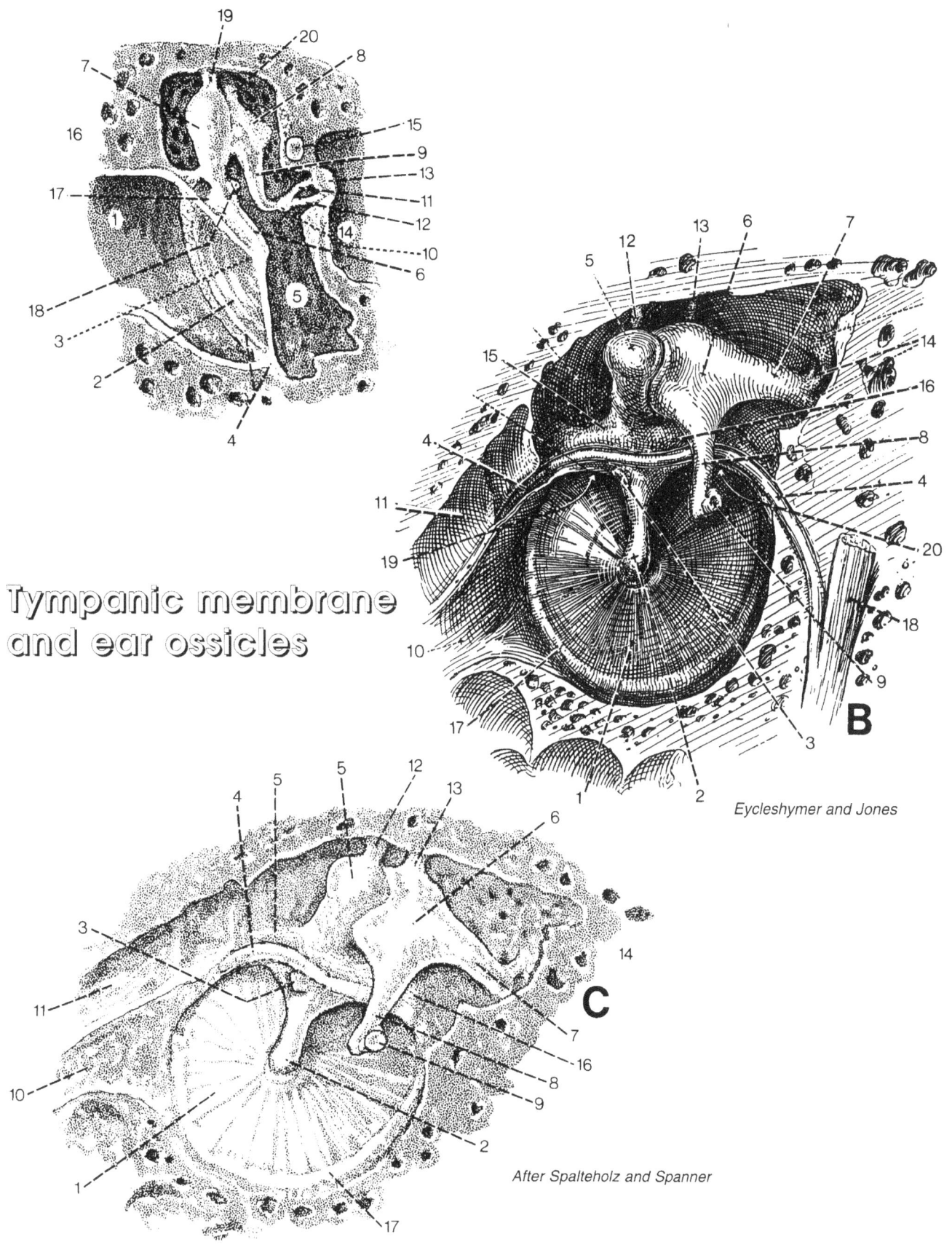

Eycleshymer and Jones

After Spalteholz and Spanner

H&N-41 Ear ossicles and part of eardrum

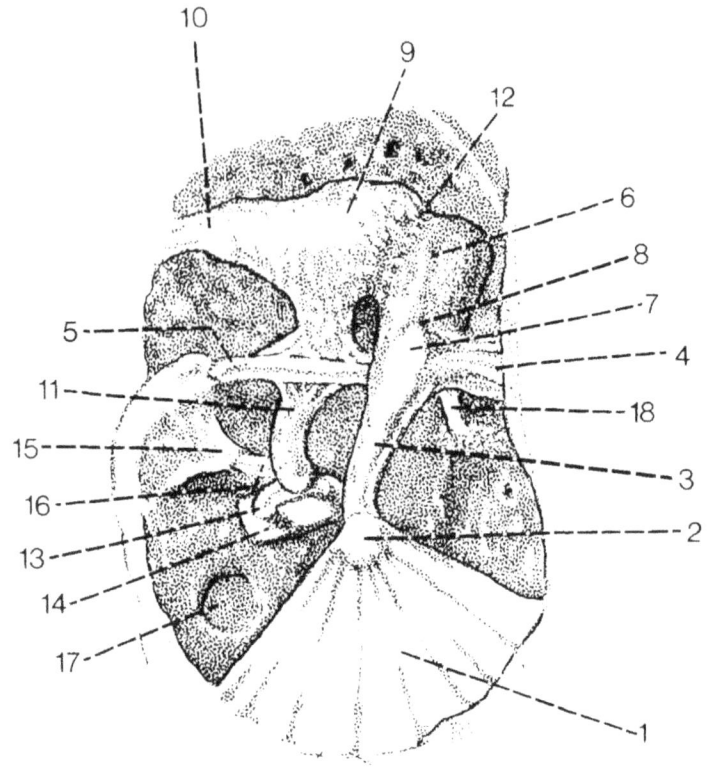

Right middle ear with eardrum largely removed. Looking in from external acoustic meatus.

Color and label

1. Tympanic membrane (eardrum; one quarter intact, three-quarters removed)
2. Umbo (note attachment of handle of malleus on inner surface of eardrum at umbo)
3. Handle of malleus
4. Anterior mallear process and ligament
5. Chorda tympani nerve (so named because of its passing adjacent to the tympanic membrane)
6. Head of malleus
7. Lateral mallear process
8. Neck of malleus
9. Body of incus
10. Short limb of incus
11. Long limb of incus
12. Incudomalleal joint
13. Stapes posterior limb
14. Footplate of stapes on oval window (fenestra vestibuli)
15. Pyramidal eminence containing stapedius muscle
16. Tendon of stapedius muscle
17. Fenestra cochleae (round window; acts as a pressure release for fluid waves in cochlea)
18. Tendon of tensor tympani muscle (acts as a damper on loud, sound-induced vibrations)

1 _____
2 _____
3 _____
4 _____
5 _____
6 _____
7 _____
8 _____
9 _____
10 _____
11 _____
12 _____
13 _____
14 _____
15 _____
16 _____
17 _____
18 _____

H&N-42 Middle ear ossicles

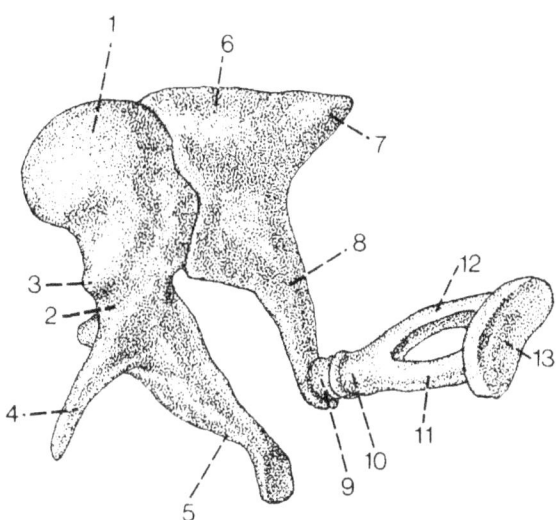

Color and label

1. Head of malleus
2. Neck of malleus
3. Lateral mallear process
4. Anterior mallear process
5. Handle of malleus
6. Body of incus
7. Short process of incus
8. Long process of incus
9. Lenticular process of incus
10. Head of stapes
11. Anterior limb (crus) of stapes
12. Posterior limb (crus) of stales
13. Footplate of stapes
14. Articular surface of malleus (with incus)
15. Articular surface of incus (with malleus)

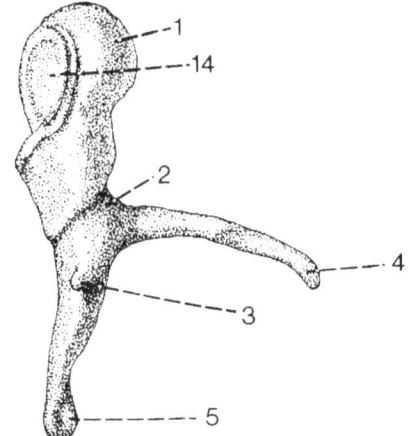

Right malleus lateral view

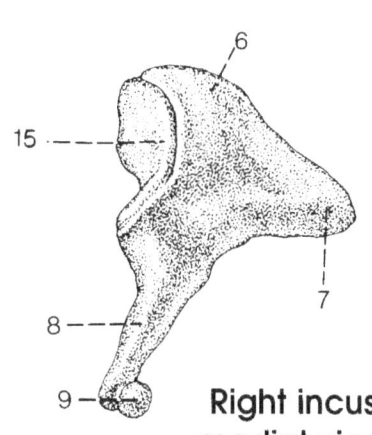

Right incus medial view

Right stapes superior view

After Wolf-Heidegger

1. _____
2. _____
3. _____
4. _____
5. _____
6. _____
7. _____
8. _____
9. _____
10. _____
11. _____
12. _____
13. _____
14. _____
15. _____

H&N-43 Dissection of right ear showing middle ear and cochlea

(opposite page)

Color and label

1. External auditory (acoustic) meatus
2. Tympanic membrane (eardrum)
3. Middle ear cavity. This is filled with air that can enter and leave only through the eustachian tube; the middle ear cavity is lined with a mucous membrane that covers its walls as well as the ear ossicles, plus that portion of the chorda tympani nerve passing through the middle ear
4. Malleus (note its handle attached to the eardrum at the umbo; sound-induced vibrations are carried across the middle ear cavity and increased in force by the three ear ossicles)
5. Incus (the three ear ossicles are joined by two synovial joints; however, the malleus and incus vibrate as a single unit; the longer length of the malleus in relation to the incus gives a leverage advantage; the end of the malleus handle moves more, whereas the shorter lenticular process end of the incus moves less but with greater force)
6. Base (footplate) of stapes on oval window (fenestra vestibuli). The eardrum is about 15 times greater in area than the footplate of the stapes. This difference in area plus the leverage advantages bestowed by the ossicles' configuration results in an increase in pressure at the oval window that is about 15 times greater than that at the eardrum.
7. Opening of vestibule into scala vestibuli. Sound-induced pressure waves from the vibrating footplate of the stapes set off fluid pressure waves in the perilymph of the vestibule which enter the scala vestibuli where they cause the membranous walls of the duct to be deflected.
8. Scala vestibuli. The snail-like conchlea is divided into three spiral compartments or scalae (Latin, staircase or ladder). The scala vestibuli and scala tympani are filled with perilymph, which has a high sodium content. The scala media, or cochlear duct, is filled with endolymph, which has a high potassium content. Arrows pointing **UP**, that is, towards the apex, indicate the course of pressure waves in the scala vestibuli.
9. Scala tympani. Arrows pointing **DOWN** indicate the course of pressure waves in the scala tympani. In cross-section the three scala each occupy the following amount of cross-section in the cochlea: scala vestibuli, about 150°; the cochlear duct, about 30°; the scala tympani, about 180°
10. Round window (now called fenestra tympani). This is covered by a membrane that moves directly opposite to the movements of the footplate of the stapes. When the footplate moves in against the perilymph in the vestibule, the membrane on the round window moves out, and vice versa. This allows the sound-induced fluid pressure waves to travel up the cochlea. Because the fluid (endolymph and perilymph) is essentially incompressible, and the cells and membrane are mainly fluid, plus the fact that the fluid-filled inner ear is encased in unyielding bone, it is essential that the membrane across the round window acts as a pressure release.
11. Cochlear duct. Filled with endolymph, it contains the organ of Corti. It is here that vibrations in the form of traveling waves in basilar membrane of the cochlear duct are transformed into nerve impulses.
12. Spiral ganglion. This consists of bipolar nerve cell bodies that supply sensory fibers to the hair cells in the organ of Corti.
13. Cochlear portion of the vestibulocochlear nerve
14. Basal turn of cochlea
15. Second turn of cochlea
16. Apex of cochlea with helicotrema, which is a small opening between the scala vestibuli and scala tympani
17. Facial nerve (N VII) (a small portion)
18. Internal auditory meatus. Contains nerves VII and VIII.
19. Facial nerve in facial canal. Note its proximity to the middle ear cavity.
20. Vestibular part of nerve VIII
21. Superior and inferior vestibular ganglia
22. Superior semicircular canal within petrous portion of temporal bone
23. Tensor tympani muscle (a portion)
24. Tendon of tensor tympani muscle. It attaches to the malleus and dampens its vibrations during loud sounds and probably during chewing and speaking.
25. Auditory (eustachian) tube. Normally it is collapsed so that air does not pass freely between the middle ear and nasopharynx. Chewing and yawning usually open the tube enough to allow air pressure in the middle ear to equalize with that of the outside air.
26. Superior petrosal sinus. A vein enclosed by dura mater
27. Temporal bone

H&N-43 Dissection of right ear showing middle ear and cochlea

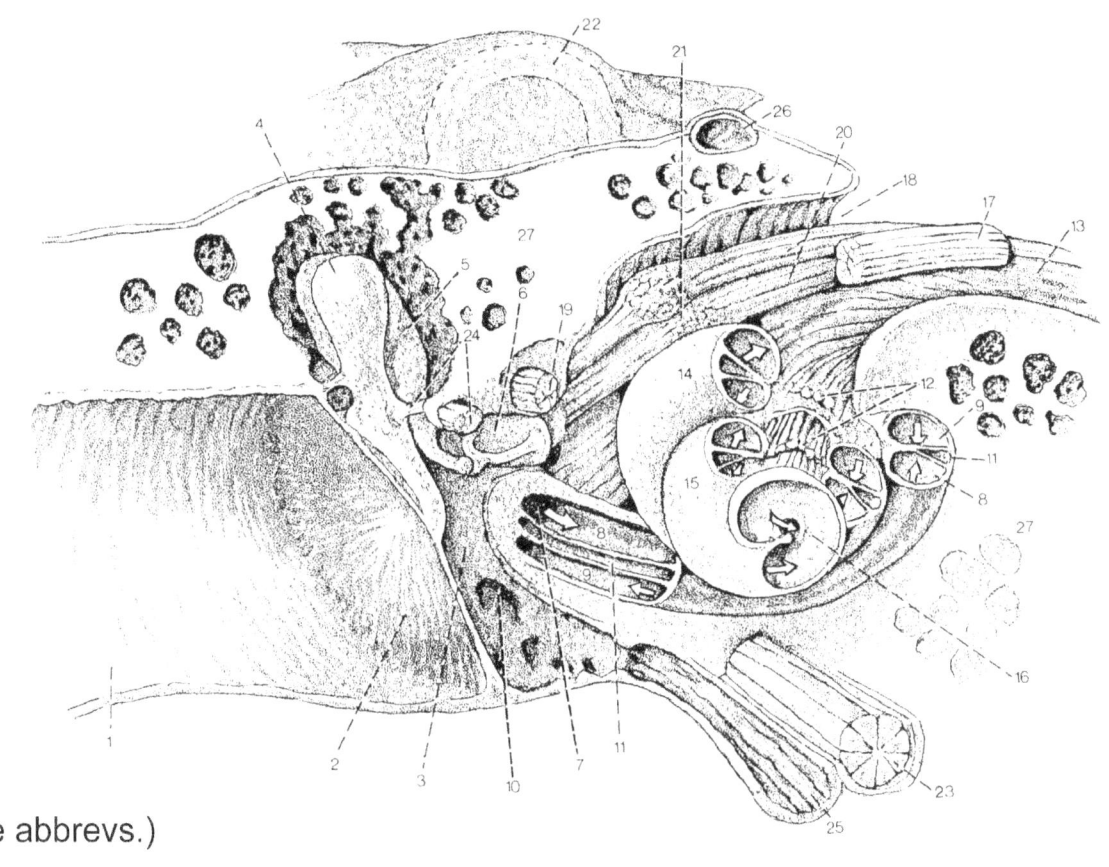

(use abbrevs.)

1 _____
2 _____
3 _____
4 _____
5 _____
6 _____
7 _____
8 _____
9 _____
10 _____
11 _____
12 _____
13 _____
14 _____
15 _____
16 _____
17 _____
18 _____
19 _____
20 _____
21 _____
22 _____
23 _____
24 _____
25 _____
26 _____
27 _____

H&N-44 Membranous labyrinth of left inner ear cut open

The membranous labyrinth lies in the bony labyrinth surrounded by perilymph.

(opposite page)

Color and label

1. Utricle (a position and motion sensor); cut open to show its continuity with each of the 3 semicircular ducts
2. Saccule. Cut open to reveal its macula. The utricle and saccule both lie in the vestibule.
3. Utricular macula. It lies mainly in a horizontal plane. Its hair cells are stimulated both by tilting the head and by accelerating and decelerating in a horizontal direction, such as speeding up and stopping suddenly in a car.
4. Saccular macula (*macula* is Latin for spot). It lies in a vertical plane and responds to vertical acceleration and deceleration, such a starting and stopping in a fast elevator.
5. Crista (L. ridge) and cupula (L. cup-shaped object) in the ampulla (L. flask) of anterior semicircular duct. The cupula in each semicircular sways in response to movement of the endolymph in the semicircular ducts.
6. Crista and cupula of lateral semicircular duct within its ampulla seen through its opening into the utricle.
7. Crista of posterior semicircular duct within it ampulla
8. Cupula on posterior crista. The three cupulae are noncellular gelatinous masses on each crista. Hair cells in the three cristae project their processes into the base of each cupula. Turning the head causes the endolymph to deflect the cupula either towards the ampulla, which fires off the hair cells, or away from the ampulla, which hyperpolarizes the air cells.
9. Utricle cut open.
10. Vestibular end of cochlear duct. This abuts on the fenestra vestibuli (round window).
11. Spiral ganglion. Its peripheral processes end in the spiral organ of Corti and its central processes form the cochlear portion of the vestibulocochlear nerve (N VIII)
12. Afferent (incoming, to the brain) nerve fibers from the bipolar neurons in the spiral ganglion. There are also some efferent (outgoing) nerve fibers.
13. Cochlear duct. Shown here without the accompanying scala vestibuli and scala tympani. The cochlear duct, or scala media, is pie-shaped in cross-section, occupying only about 30 degress of the cross-section of the cochlea.
14. Anterior semicircular duct. Each semicircular duct lies within a semicircular canal.
15. Lateral semicircular duct
16. Posterior semicircular duct
17. Endolymphatic duct. Its enlarged end lies adjacent to the dura mater.
18. Nerve to posterior crista ampullaris
19. Upper division of vestibular nerve
20. Lower division of vestibular nerve
21. Cochlear nerve

Vertigo (Latin, *vertere,* to turn): a feeling of whirling or turning around, a giddiness, a dizziness. An hallucination of movement, expecially of rotation, independent of any actual movement. Vestibular vertigo, such as occurs in Meniere's disease, is due to disease within the vestibular labyrinth, which includes the three semicircular ducts, the utricle, and the saccule.

H&N-44 Membranous labyrinth of left inner ear cut open
Removed from bony labyrinth and partially dissected

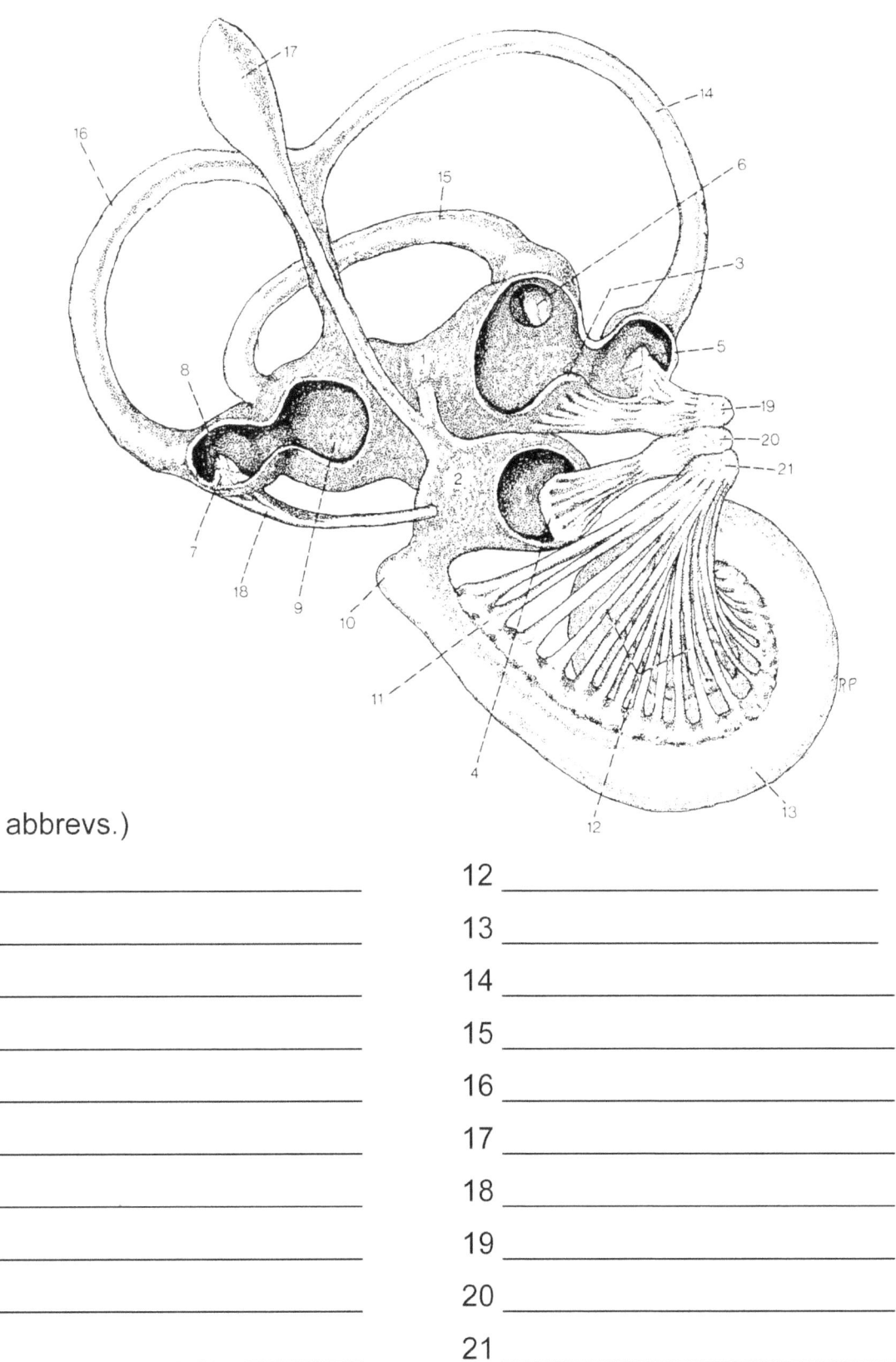

(use abbrevs.)

1 _____
2 _____
3 _____
4 _____
5 _____
6 _____
7 _____
8 _____
9 _____
10 _____
11 _____

12 _____
13 _____
14 _____
15 _____
16 _____
17 _____
18 _____
19 _____
20 _____
21 _____

H&N-45 Dissection of right temporal bone showing sigmoid sinus and facial canal

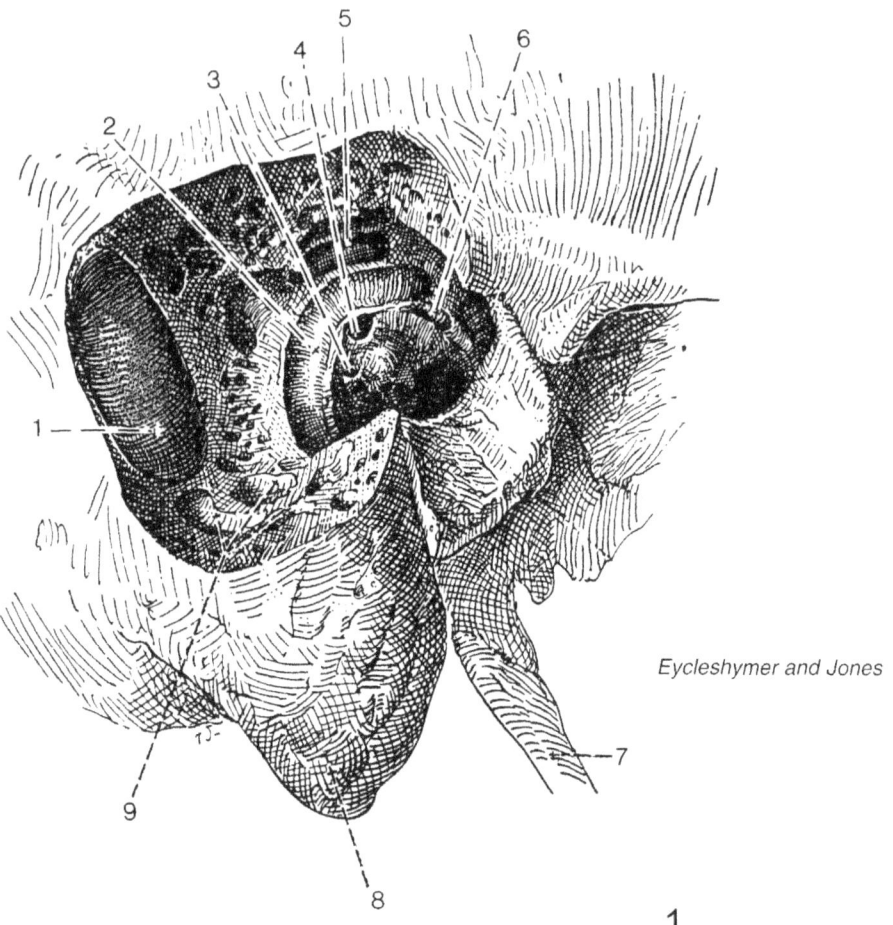

Eycleshymer and Jones

Color and label

1. Sigmoid sinus; directly continuous with transverse sinus; becomes the internal jugular vein upon leaving the skull via the jugular foramen
2. Facial canal
3. Round window
4. Oval window; covered by footplate of stapes
5. Lateral semicircular canal
6. Canal for tensor tympani muscle
7. Styloid process
8. Mastoid process (breast-like, *mastos*, Greek, breast)
9. Mastoid air cells

1 _____
2 _____
3 _____
4 _____
5 _____
6 _____
7 _____
8 _____
9 _____

H&N-46 Section through external ear, middle ear, and inner ear

Color and label

1 Helix of auricle (external ear)*
2 Antihelix of auricle*
3 Concha of auricle*
4 External acoustic (auditory) meatus (cartilaginous part)
5 Mastoid process
6 Ear drum (tympanic membrane)
7 Head of stapes
8 Tympanic cavity (cavity of middle ear)
9 Levator veli palatini muscle
10 Superior pharyngeal constrictor muscle
11 External auditory meatus (bony part)
12 Epitympanic recess
13 Head of malleus
14 Anterior semicircular duct (within anterior semicircular canal)
15 Utricle
16 Endolymphatic duct
17 Sacculus; both the saccule and the utricle occupy the vestibule, a small cavity in the temporal bone
18 Tensor tympani muscle
19 Cochlear duct
20 Tympanic opening of the auditory tube (old name, Eustachean tube)
21 Bony part of auditory tube
22 Isthmus of auditory tube
23 Cartilage of auditory tube
24 Cartilaginous part of auditory tube
25 Pharyngeal opening of auditory tube

Somewhat diagrammatic

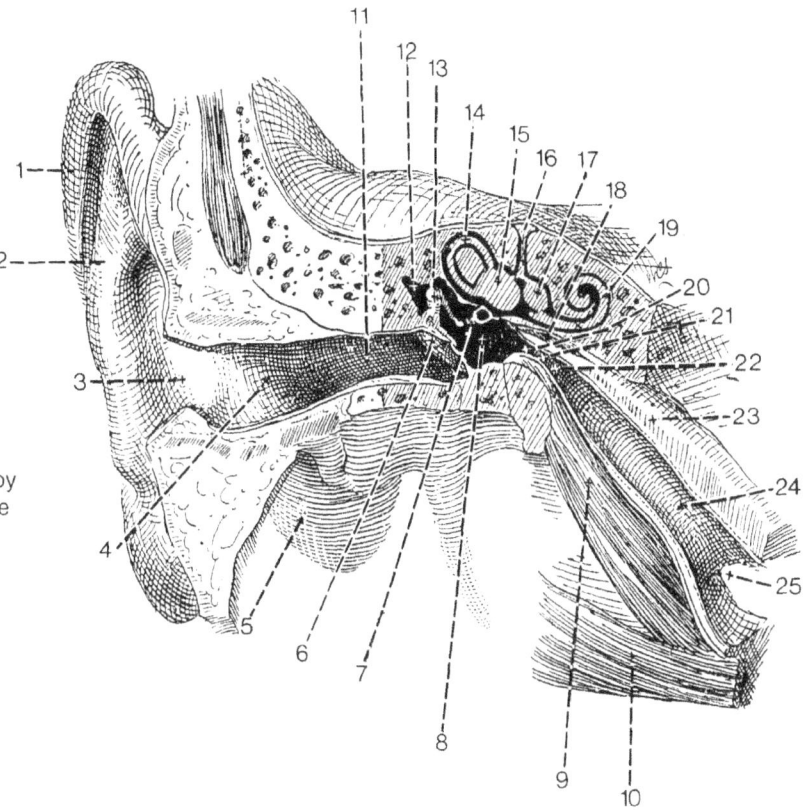

Eycleshymer and Jones with slight modification

*The Terminologia Anatomica lists 29 anatomical parts of the auricle of the ear, only three of which are identified here.

1 _____	14 _____
2 _____	15 _____
3 _____	16 _____
4 _____	17 _____
5 _____	18 _____
6 _____	19 _____
7 _____	20 _____
8 _____	21 _____
9 _____	22 _____
10 _____	23 _____
11 _____	24 _____
12 _____	25 _____
13 _____	

Tragus
Etymological cartoon

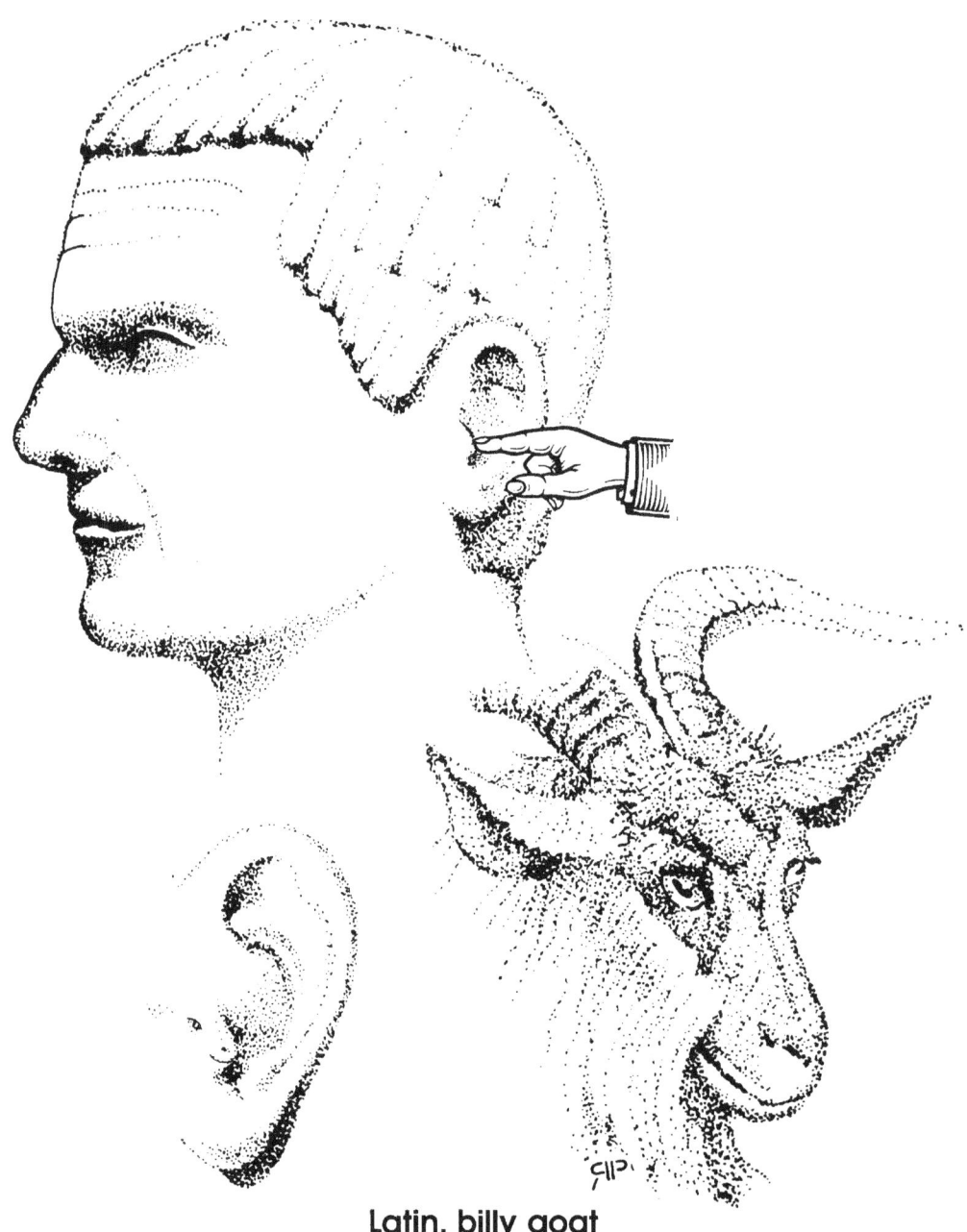

Latin, billy goat

The tragus of the ear was so named because in some old men it grows a little tuft of hair that reminded the ancient anatomists of a billy goat's beard. Tragos is Greek for billy goat and tragus is the Latin. Tragedy originally meant "goat's song."

H&N-47 Cartilages of the nose

Color and label
1. Greater alar cartilage
2. Lateral crus of greater alar cartilage
3. Medial crus of greater alar cartilage
4. Lateral nasal cartilage
5. Accessory nasal cartilage
6. Minor alar cartilage
7. Nasal septal cartilage
8. Nasal bone
9. Maxillary bone

1 _____
2 _____
3 _____
4 _____
5 _____
6 _____
7 _____
8 _____
9 _____

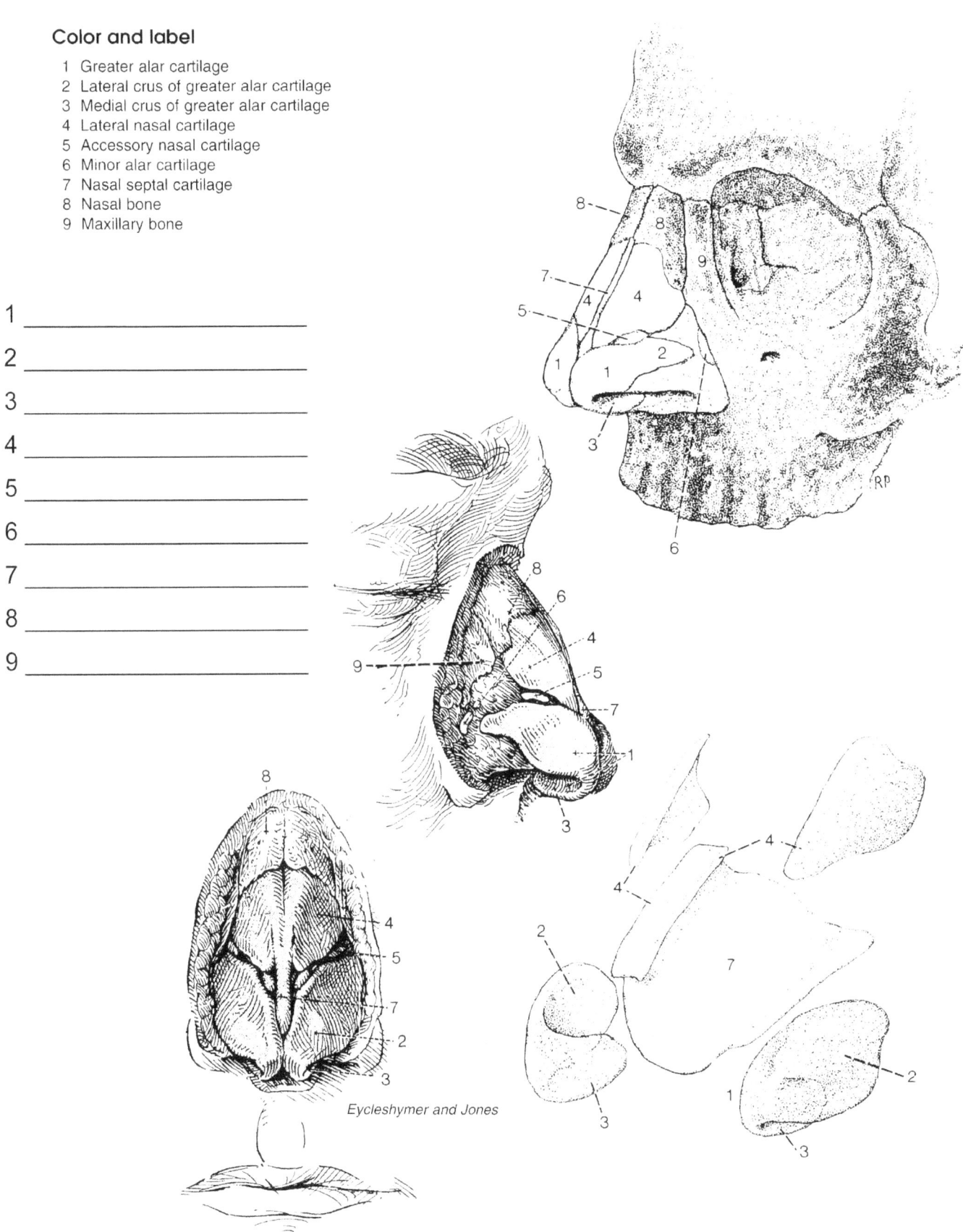

Eycleshymer and Jones

H&N-48 Nasal cavity, lateral wall

Right nasal cavity: conchae cut* in lower figure

Color and label

1. Superior nasal concha*
2. Middle nasal concha*
3. Inferior nasal concha*
4. Frontal sinus
5. Crista galli (not to be confused with Crystal Gale; *crista galli* is Latin for rooster's comb)*
6. Sphenoidal sinus
7. Opening of sphenoidal sinus
8. Superior nasal meatus
9. Middle nasal meatus
10. Inferior nasal meatus
11. Opening of auditory tube in nasal pharynx
12. Hard palate
13. Soft palate

*Crystal Gale is a country blues singer. Although crista galli and Cristal Gale sound alike, they don't at all look alike.

14. Agger nasi (*agger*, Latin, mound)
15. Pharyngeal tonsil (called adenoids when inflamed)
16. Ethmoidal bulla (Latin, swelling)
17. Openings of ethmoidal air cells
18. Hiatus semilunaris
19. Opening of frontal sinus into hiatus semilunaris
20. Opening of nasolacrimal duct into inferior nasal meatus

21. Opening of maxillary sinus into hiatus semilunaris
22. Spheno-ethmoidal recess
23. Nasal vestibule
24. Choana (posterior opening of nasal cavity into nasal pharynx)
25. Probe in opening of sphenoidal sinus
26. Nasal pharynx (also, nasopharynx)

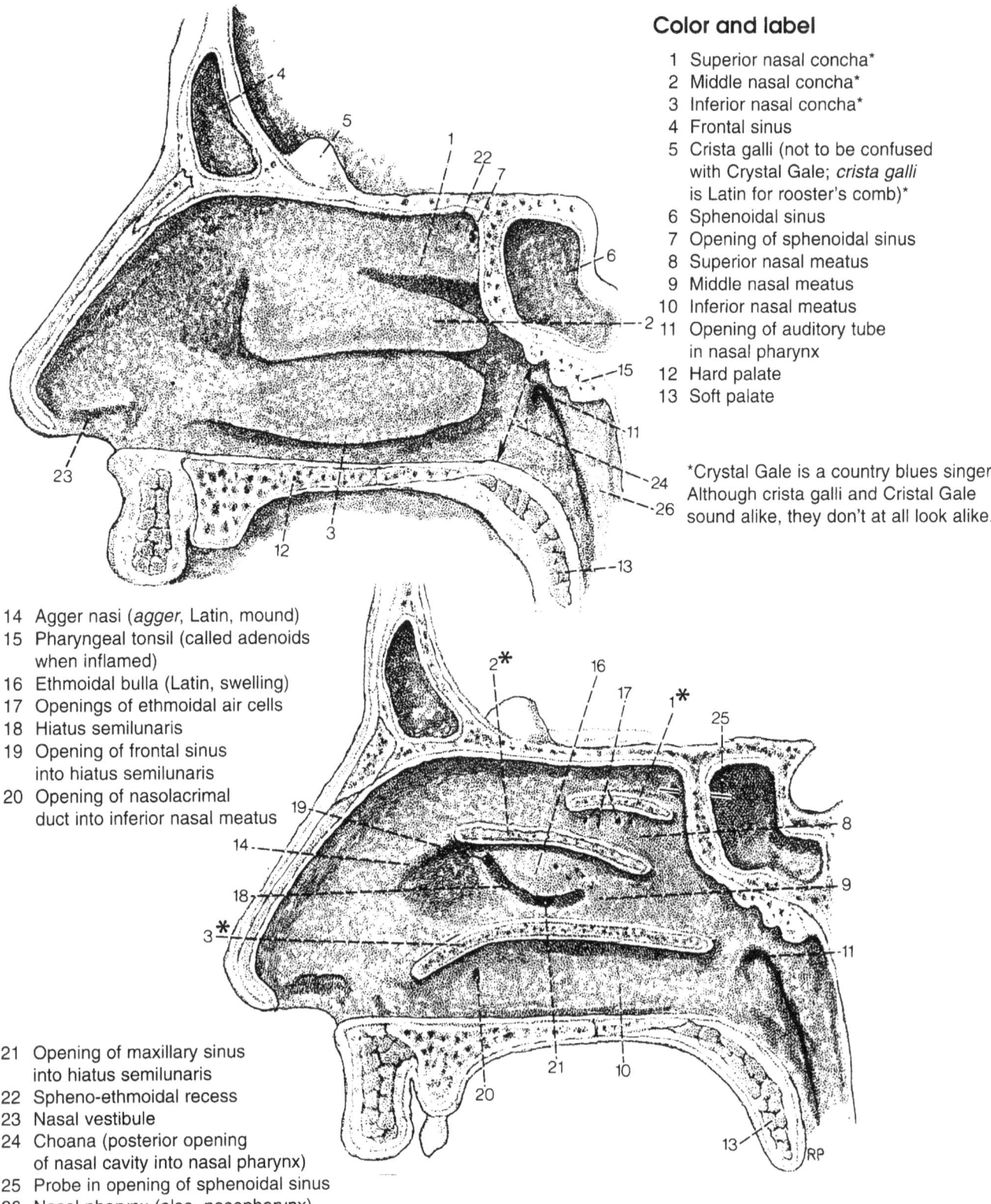

H&N-48 Nasal cavity, lateral wall

Right nasal cavity: conchae cut* in lower figure

1 _____
2 _____
3 _____
4 _____
5 _____
6 _____
7 _____
8 _____
9 _____
10 _____
11 _____
12 _____
13 _____
14 _____
15 _____
16 _____
17 _____
18 _____
19 _____
20 _____
21 _____
22 _____
23 _____
24 _____
25 _____
26 _____

H&N-49 Nasal cavity, bones and cartilages

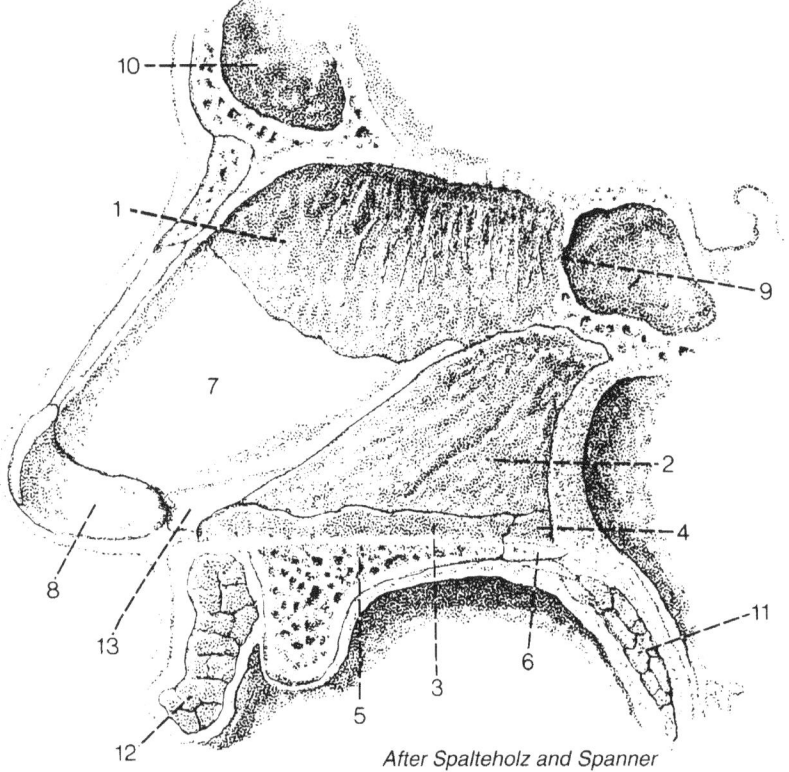

After Spalteholz and Spanner

Color and label

1. Perpendicular plate of ethmoid bone
2. Vomer (Latin, plowshare)
3. Nasal spine of maxillary bone
4. Nasal spine of palatine bone
5. Palatine process of maxilla
6. Horizontal plate of palatine bone
7. Nasal septal cartilage
8. Left greater alar cartilage (medial crus) (cut; with lateral crus removed)
9. Sphenoidal sinus and opening
10. Frontal sinus
11. Soft palate
12. Upper lip
13. Vomeronasal cartilage

Right side of nasal cavity

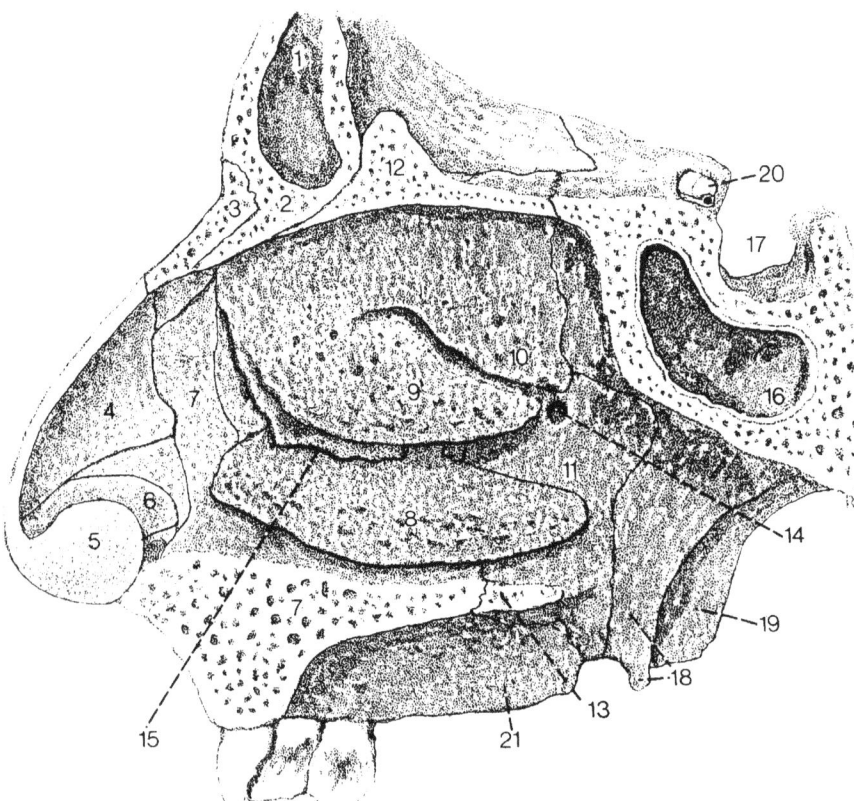

1. Frontal sinus
2. Frontal bone
3. Nasal bone
4. Lateral nasal cartilage
5. Greater alar cartilage (medial crus)
6. Greater alar cartilage (lateral crus)
7. Maxillary bone
8. Inferior nasal concha (a separate bone)
9. Middle nasal concha (part of the ethmoid bone)
10. Superior nasal concha (part of ethmoid bone)
11. Palatine bone (vertical part)
12. Crista galli (part of ethmoid)
13. Palatine bone (horizontal part)
14. Sphenopalatine foramen
15. Uncinate process (part of ethmoid)
16. Sphenoidal sinus
17. Hypophyseal fossa
18. Medial pterygoid plate (part of sphenoid bone)
19. Lateral pterygoid plate (part of sphenoid bone)
20. Optic nerve and ophthalmic artery
21. Alveolar process of maxillary bone

H&N-49 Nasal cavity, bones and cartilages
(opposite page)

1 _____
2 _____
3 _____
4 _____
5 _____
6 _____
7 _____

8 _____
9 _____
10 _____
11 _____
12 _____
13 _____

Right side of nasal cavity

1 _____
2 _____
3 _____
4 _____
5 _____
6 _____
7 _____
8 _____
9 _____
10 _____
11 _____

12 _____
13 _____
14 _____
15 _____
16 _____
17 _____
18 _____
19 _____
20 _____
21 _____

H&N-50 Nasal cavity, lateral wall and frontal section

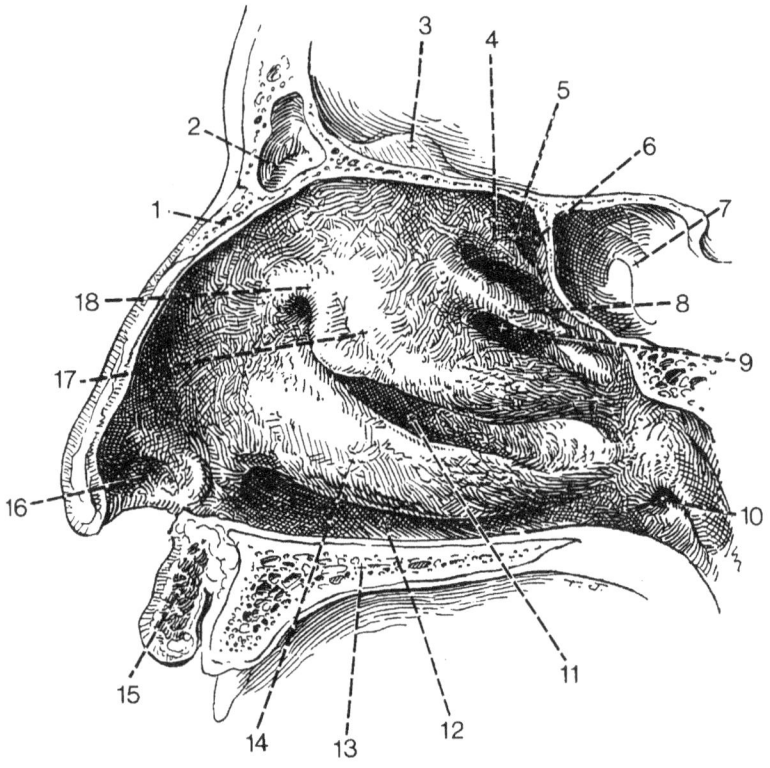

Right lateral wall

Color and label

1. Nasal bone
2. Frontal sinus
3. Crista galli
4. Supreme nasal concha
5. Spheno-ethmoidal recess
6. Opening of sphenoidal sinus
7. Sphenoidal sinus
8. Superior nasal concha
9. Superior nasal meatus
10. Pharyngeal opening of auditory tube
11. Middle nasal meatus
12. Inferior nasal meatus
13. Hard palate (horizontal plate of maxillary bone)
14. Inferior nasal concha
15. Superior lip (Latin, *labium superius*)
16. Vestibule of the nose
17. Middle nasal concha
18. Agger nasi (*agger*, Latin, heap, mound, rampart)
19. Anterior ethmoidal air cell
20. Ethmoidal bulla (bulla, Latin, a bubble-like protuberance)
21. Uncinate process (uncinate, hook-shaped)
22. Maxillary sinus
23. Septum of nose
24. Eye in orbit
25. Arrow passing through maxillary sinus opening

Frontal section

Eycleshymer and Jones

H&N-50 Nasal cavity, lateral wall and frontal section
(opposite page)

1 _____
2 _____
3 _____
4 _____
5 _____
6 _____
7 _____
8 _____
9 _____
10 _____
11 _____
12 _____
13 _____

14 _____
15 _____
16 _____
17 _____
18 _____
19 _____
20 _____
21 _____
22 _____
23 _____
24 _____
25 _____

H&N-51 Pterygopalatine ganglion

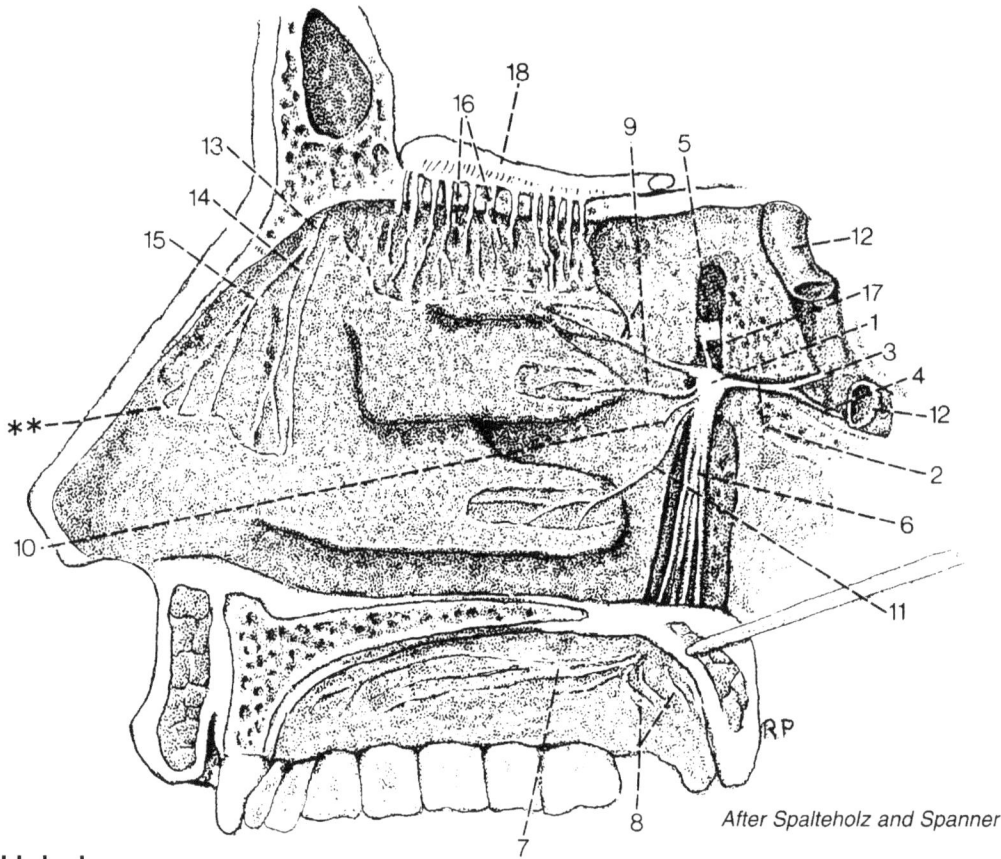

After Spalteholz and Spanner

Color and label

1. Pterygopalatine ganglion*; contains postganglionic parasympathetic neurons with secretomotor axons destined for the posterior nasal glands and lacrimal gland; only pregangionic parasympathetic axons synapse within this ganglion, other fibers bypass it.
2. Nerve of the pterygoid canal; made up of the greater petrosal (taste and parasympatheic fibers from the facial nerve) and the deep petrosal nerve (sympathetic fibers from cell bodies in the superior cervical ganglion).
3. Greater petrosal nerve
4. Deep petrosal nerve
5. Maxillary in the pterygopalatine fossa*
6. Palatine nerves; descending in palatine canal*
7. Greater palatine nerves
8. Lesser palatine nerves
9. Lateral superior posterior nasal branches of maxillary nerve and pterygopalatine ganglion
10. Medial superior posterior nasal branches to nasal septum from maxillary nerve and pterygopalatine ganglion (cut)
11. Lateral inferior posterior nasal branches of maxillary nerve and pterygopalatine ganglion
12. Internal carotid artery (cut both entering [bottom], and leaving [top] the cavernous sinus)
13. Internal nasal branches of anterior ethmoidal nerve of ophthalmic nerve
14. Lateral nasal branches
15. External nasal branches
16. Olfactory nerves (cranial nerve I; note axons ending in olfactory bulb after passing through cribriform [sieve-like, full of holes] plate of ethmoid bone)
17. Pterygopalatine nerves
18. Olfactory bulb

*Pterygopalatine fossa and palatine canal opened from medial aspect

**Mucous membrane removed to display nerves

H&N-51 Pterygopalatine ganglion

(opposite page)

1 _____
2 _____
3 _____
4 _____
5 _____
6 _____
7 _____
8 _____
9 _____
10 _____
11 _____
12 _____
13 _____
14 _____
15 _____
16 _____
17 _____
18 _____

H&N-52 Olfactory nerves and arterial supply of nasal cavity

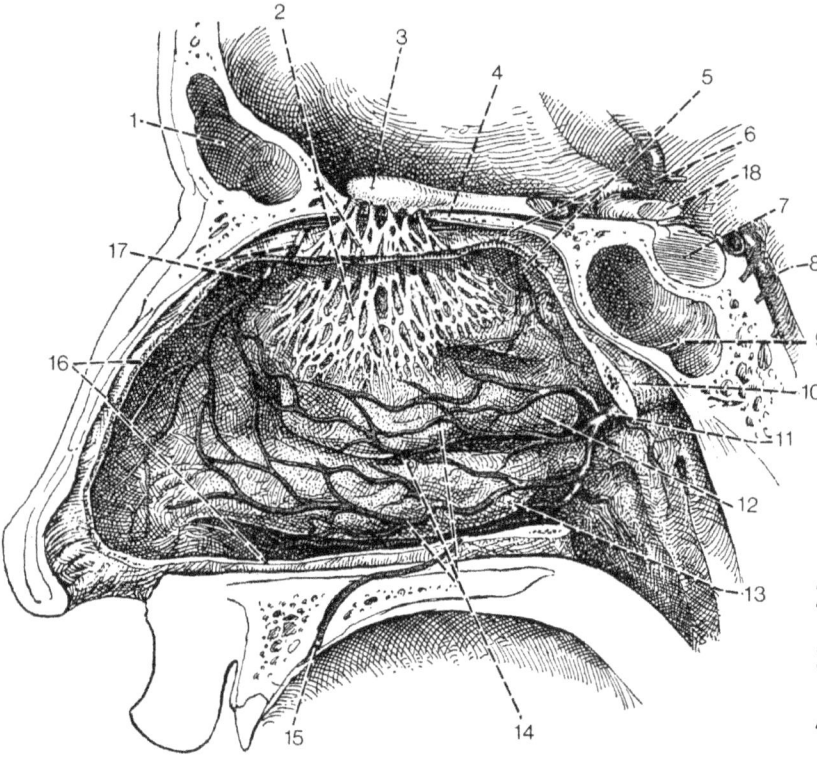

Color and label

Eycleshymer and Jones

1. Frontal sinus
2. Olfactory nerves (cranial nerve I); note their passing through the cribriform plate; note also olfactory nerves on the nasal septum (where both septum and nerves are cut)
3. Olfactory bulb; compared to mammals such as dogs, humans have relatively small olfactory bulbs and rely largely on vision, rather than olfaction, for perceiving our surroundings. (Macrosmatic means having a well-developed olfactory sense; microsmatic means having a poorly developed olfactory sense; *osme*, Greek, smell.)
4. Cribriform plate of ethmoid bone
5. Posterior ethmoidal artery; including cut branch on nasal septum (also cut)
6. Internal carotid artery
7. Hypophysis (pituitary gland)
8. Basilar artery
9. Sphenoid sinus
10. Nasal septum (posterior part; cut)
11. Sphenopalatine artery
12. Middle nasal concha
13. Inferior nasal concha
14. Lateral posterior nasal arteries
15. Artery in incisive canal (anastomosis between septal nasal artery and greater palatine artery)
16. Nasal septum (cut)
17. Anterior ethmoidal artery
18. Optic nerve (cranial nerve II; cut)

H&N-53 Right wall of nasal cavity and ethmoidal air cells

The middle and superior conchae have been removed.

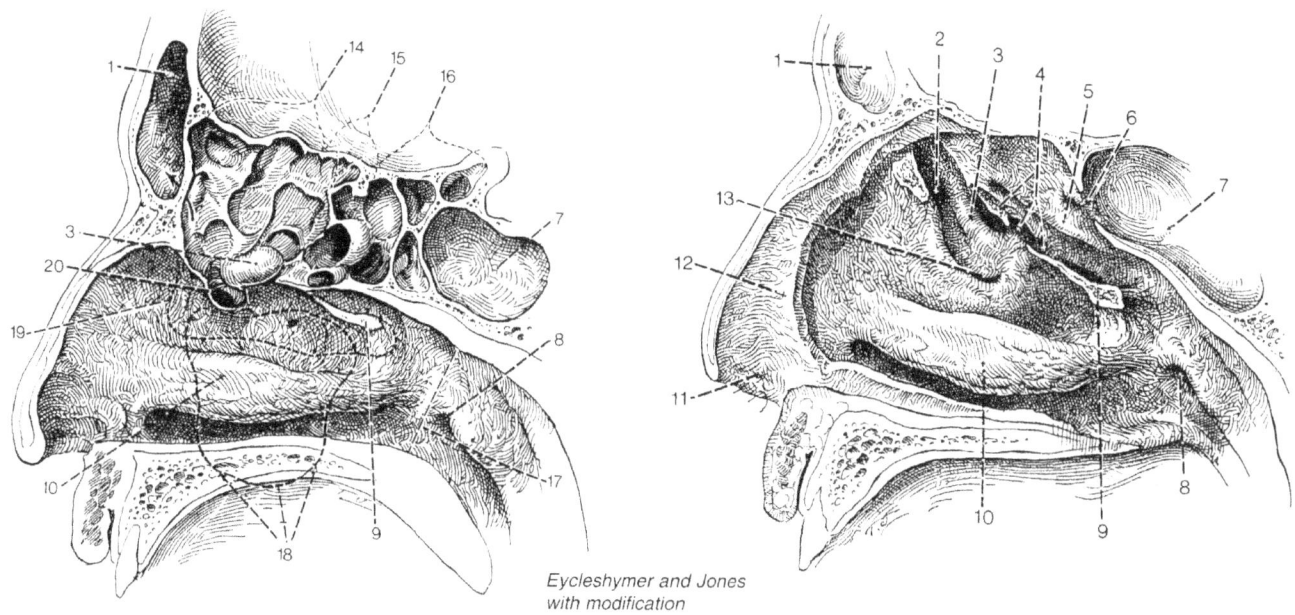

Eycleshymer and Jones with modification

1 _____   11 _____
2 _____   12 _____
3 _____   13 _____
4 _____   14 _____
5 _____   15 _____
6 _____   16 _____
7 _____   17 _____
8 _____   18 _____
9 _____   19 _____
10 _____   20 _____

Color and label

1 Frontal sinus
2 Ethmoidal infundibulum
3 Ethmoidal bulla
4 Superior nasal concha (cut and removed) and superior nasal meatus
5 Highest (supreme) nasal concha
6 Opening of sphenoidal sinus
7 Sphenoidal sinus; note the variation in both size and shape in the frontal and sphenoidal sinuses in the two figures.
8 Pharyngeal opening of the auditory tube
9 Middle nasal concha (cut and removed)
10 Inferior nasal concha
11 Nasal vestibule
12 Nasal septum (cut and largely removed)
13 Hiatus semilunaris
14 Anterior ethmoidal (air) cells
15 Middle ethmoidal (air) cells
16 Posterior ethmoidal (air) cells
17 Posterior nasal aperature (or choana)
18 Projected outline of maxillary sinus
19 Outline of middle nasal concha (cut and removed)
20 Opening into maxillary sinus

H&N-54 Projection of paranasal sinuses on front and side of face

Eycleshymer and Jones

1 _____
2 _____
3 _____
4 _____
5 _____
6 _____
7 _____
8 _____
9 _____
10 _____

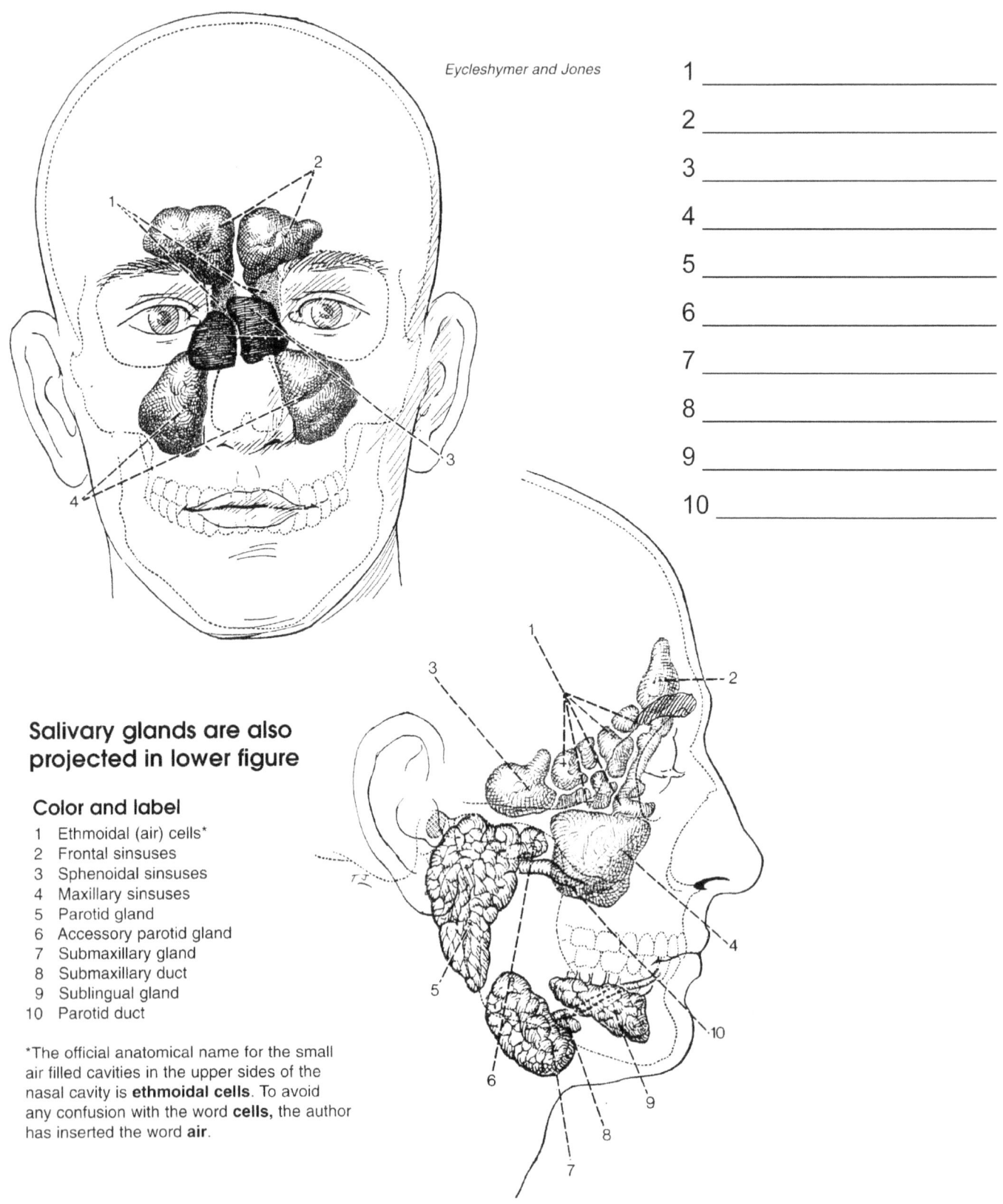

Salivary glands are also projected in lower figure

Color and label
1 Ethmoidal (air) cells*
2 Frontal sinuses
3 Sphenoidal sinsuses
4 Maxillary sinsuses
5 Parotid gland
6 Accessory parotid gland
7 Submaxillary gland
8 Submaxillary duct
9 Sublingual gland
10 Parotid duct

*The official anatomical name for the small air filled cavities in the upper sides of the nasal cavity is **ethmoidal cells**. To avoid any confusion with the word **cells,** the author has inserted the word **air**.

H&N-55 Oral and nasal cavities in sagittal section

Eycleshymer and Jones

1 _____
2 _____
3 _____
4 _____
5 _____
6 _____
7 _____
8 _____
9 _____
10 _____
11 _____
12 _____
13 _____
14 _____
15 _____
16 _____
17 _____

Color and label

1 Hard palate
2 Inferior nasal concha
3 Middle nasal concha
4 Torus tubularis (tubal prominence; *torus*, Latin, raised ridge, bulge); the protuberance of the base of cartilaginous part of the auditory tube in the lateral wall of the nasopharynx behind the orifice of the auditory tube.
5 Sphenoidal sinus
6 Pharyngeal orifice (opening) of auditory tube
7 Pharyngeal tonsil; usually absent in adults (the term *adenoids* denotes hypertrophy of this tonsil)
8 Pharyngeal recess
9 Salpingopharyngeal fold
10 Anterior arch of first cervical vertebra (atlas)
11 Soft palate
12 Second cervical vertebra (axis)
13 Palatopharyngeal arch
14 Palatine tonsil
15 Palatoglossal arch
16 Dorsum of tongue
17 White arrow indicates right choana (posterior nasal aperature; *choana*, Latin, a funnel); the two choanae are oval openings connecting each nasal cavity with the nasal pharynx.

H&N-56 Skull, coronal section
(opposite page)

1 _____
2 _____
3 _____
4 _____
5 _____
6 _____
7 _____
8 _____
9 _____
10 _____
11 _____
12 _____
13 _____
14 _____
15 _____
16 _____
17 _____
18 _____

H&N-56 Skull, coronal section

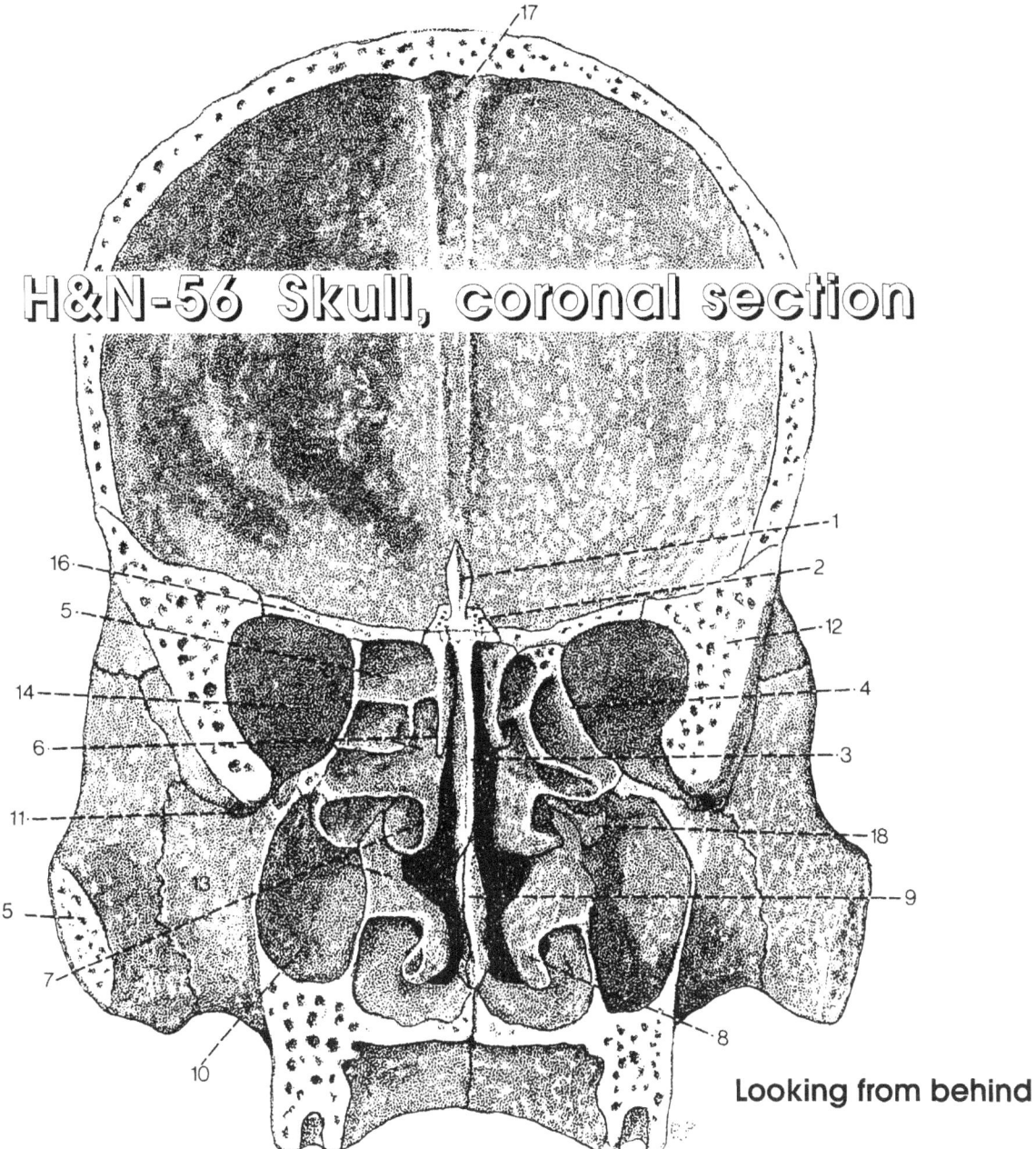

Looking from behind

Color and label

1. Crista galli (Latin, rooster's crest; part of ethmoid)
2. Cribriform (Latin, sieve-like) plate of ethmoid (contains foramina for olfactory nerves)
3. Perpendicular plate of ethmoid
4. Orbital plate of ethmoid (formerly called *lamina papyraceus* because to the ancient anatomists it was as thin as papyrus paper)
5. Ethmoidal air cells (these number 3-18 on each side)
6. Superior nasal concha (Latin, seashell; part of ethmoid) and superior nasal meatus (the passage immediately below it)
7. Middle nasal concha (part of ethmoid) and middle nasal meatus
8. Inferior nasal concha (a separate bone) and inferior nasal meatus
9. Vomer (Latin, plowshare)
10. Maxillary sinus
11. Inferior orbital fissure
12. Greater wing of sphenoid bone
13. Maxillary bone (or maxilla)
14. Orbit
15. Zygomatic bone (zygomatic arch cut)
16. Orbital part of frontal bone
17. Groove for superior sagittal sinus
18. Uncinate (Latin, hook-like) process of ethmoid

After Spalteholz and Spanner

H&N-57 Sagittal section of head

(opposite page)

Color and label

1. Crista galli
2. Cribriform plate of ethmoid bone
3. Superior nasal concha
4. Sphenoidal sinus
5. Hypophysis (pituitary gland)
6. Pharnygeal opening of auditory tube
7. Torus tubularis (bump caused by auditory tube)
8. Soft palate
9. Foramen cecum of tongue
10. Dens (odontoid process) of axis (C2)
11. Root of tongue
12. Oral part of pharynx (lower border of soft palate to level of hyoid bone)
13. Laryngeal part of pharynx (hyoid bone to lower border of cricoid cartilage)*
14. Epiglottis
15. Transverse arytenoid muscle
16. Lamina of cricoid cartilage
17. Vocal folds (true vocal cords)
18. Esophagus
19. Trachea
20. Brachiocephalic vein (old name, innominate vein)
21. Brachiocephalic artery (old name, innominate artery)
22. Frontal sinus
23. Nasal bone
24. Middle nasal concha
25. Inferior nasal concha
26. Hard palate
27. Upper lip
28. Body of tongue
29. Lower lip
30. Septum of tongue
31. Genioglossus muscle
32. Mandible
33. Geniohyoid muscle
34. Mylohyoid muscle
35. Hyoid bone
36. Vestibule of larynx
37. Thyroid cartilage
38. Arch of cricoid cartilage
39. Sternohyoid muscle
40. Thyroid gland
41. Sternothyroid gland
42. Manubrium of sternum (*manubrium*, Latin, handle)

White arrow: right choana (Greek, afunnel): the paired openings between the nasal cavity and the nasopharynx

1 _____ 22 _____
2 _____ 23 _____
3 _____ 24 _____
4 _____ 25 _____
5 _____ 26 _____
6 _____ 27 _____
7 _____ 28 _____
8 _____ 29 _____
9 _____ 30 _____
10 _____ 31 _____
11 _____ 32 _____
12 _____ 33 _____
13 _____ 34 _____
14 _____ 35 _____
15 _____ 36 _____
16 _____ 37 _____
17 _____ 38 _____
18 _____ 39 _____
19 _____ 40 _____
20 _____ 41 _____
21 _____ 42 _____

*The nasal part of the pharynx lies posterior to the nasal cavities above the soft palate. Unlike the oral and laryngeal parts, which temporarily close during swollowing, the nasal part of the pharynx (or nasopharynx) always remains open.

H&N-57 Sagittal section of head

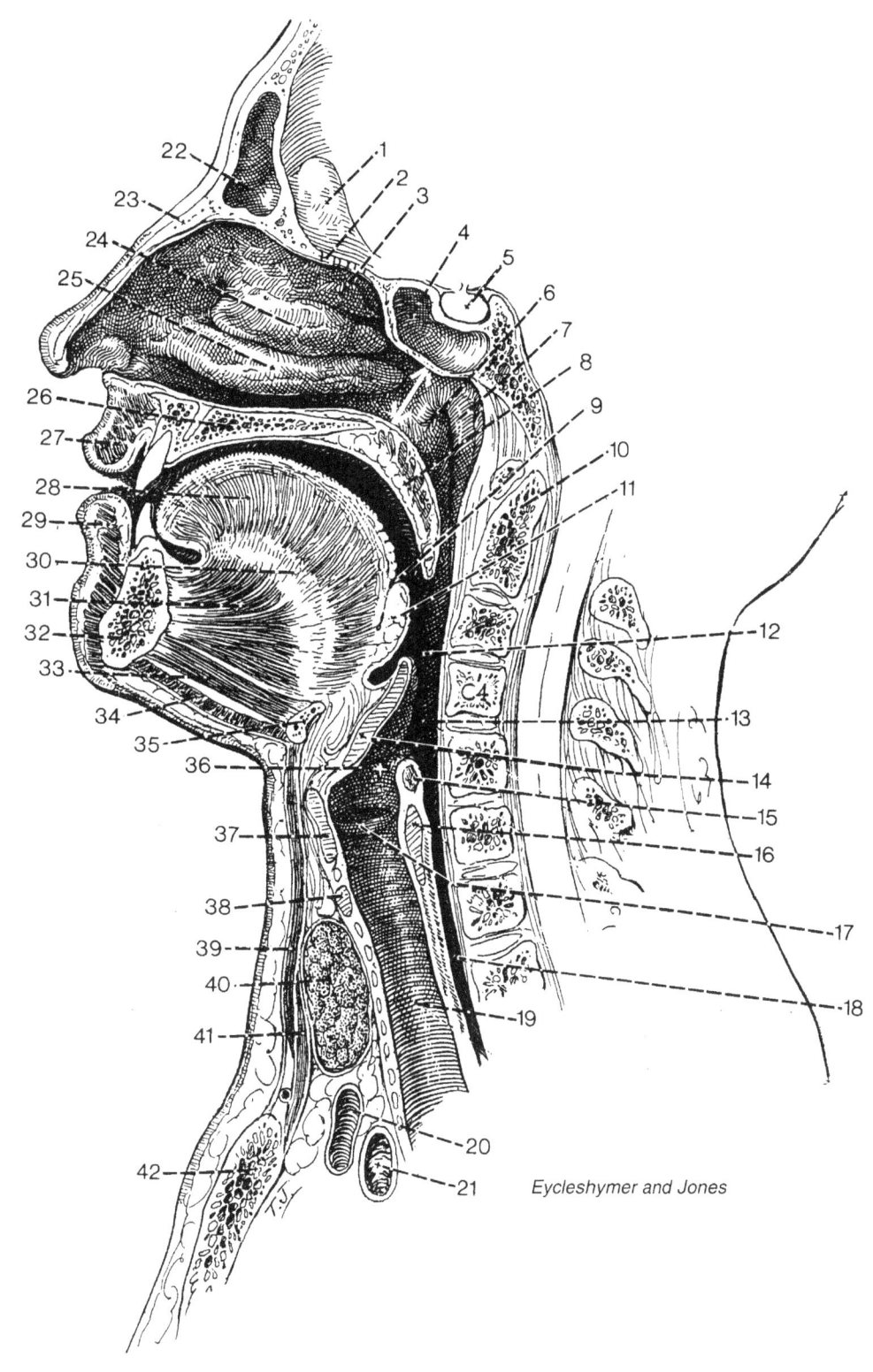

Eycleshymer and Jones

H&N-58 Pharynx

Viewed from behind. Posterior wall has been cut and retracted.

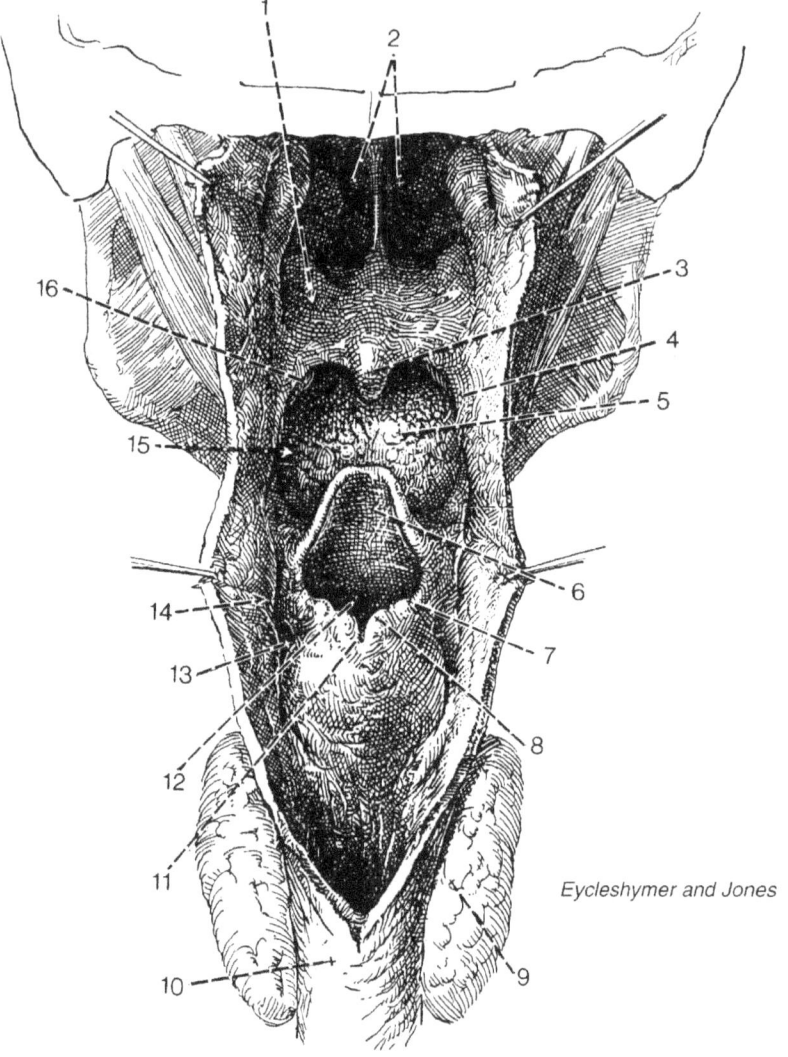

Eycleshymer and Jones

Color and label

1. Nasal part of pharynx (extends to lower edge of soft palate)
2. Choanae (two posterior openings of nasal cavity into nasal pharynx)
3. Uvula (Latin, little grape) of the soft palate
4. Palatopharyngeal arch
5. Root of tongue (pain, touch, temperature, and taste supplied by glossopharyngeal nerve)
6. Epiglottis; this covers the opening to the larynx when swallowing.
7. Cuneiform tubercle (caused by the underlying cuneiform cartilage)
8. Corniculate tubercle (caused by the underlying corniculate cartilage)
9. Thyroid gland
10. Esophagus
11. Interarytenoid incisure (*incisura*, Latin, a cut, a groove); a small notch between the two corniculate cartilages and the apices of the arytenoid cartilages on the posterior aditus of the larynx.
12. Aditus (opening) to the larynx
13. Piriform recess; a site where foreign bodies may lodge and abscesses may develope.
14. Laryngeal part of pharynx; extends from level of hyoid bone to lower border of cricoid cartilage.
15. Oral part of pharynx; extends from lower border of soft palate to level of hyoid bone.
16. Palatine tonsil

1 _____
2 _____
3 _____
4 _____
5 _____
6 _____
7 _____
8 _____
9 _____
10 _____
11 _____
12 _____
13 _____
14 _____
15 _____
16 _____

H&N-59 Muscles of the tongue, pharynx, and larynx

Right side

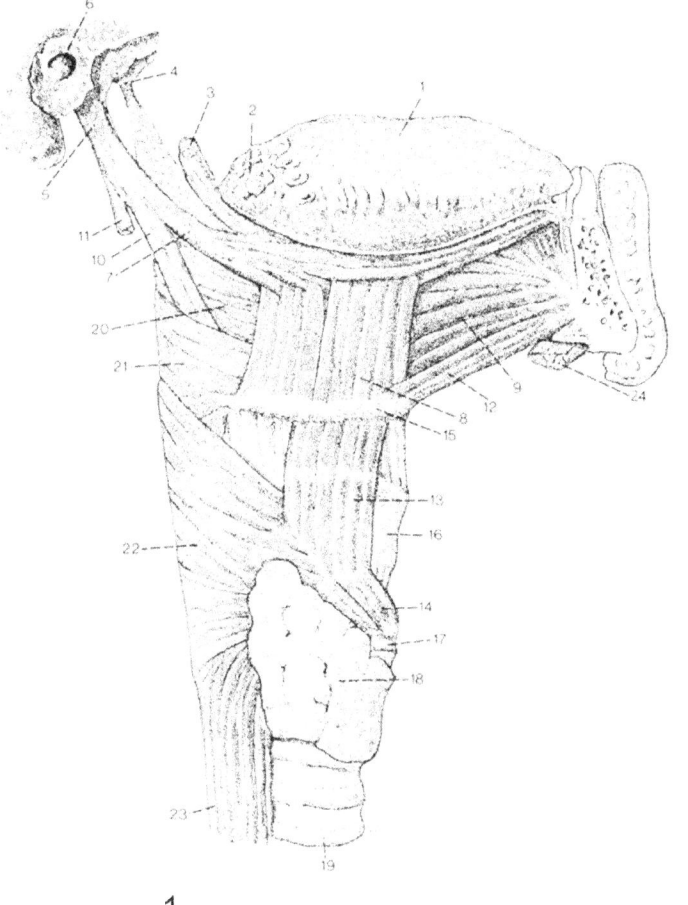

Color and label

1. Dorsum of tongue (superior visible surface)
2. Root of tongue containing lingual follicles
3. Palatoglossal muscle (cut)
4. Pharyngeal tubercle (cranial attachment of pharyngobasilar fascia)
5. Styloid process
6. External auditory meatus
7. Styloglossus muscle (innervated by hypoglossal nerve)
8. Hyoglossus muscle (innervated by hypoglossal nerve)
9. Genioglossus muscle (innervated by hypoglossal nerve)
10. Stylopharyngeus muscle (only muscle innervated solely by glossopharyngeal nerve)
11. Stylohyoid muscle (cut; innervated by facial nerve)
12. Geniohyoid muscle
13. Thyrohyoid muscle
14. Cricothyroid muscle
15. Hyoid bone
16. Thyroid cartilage
17. Cricoid cartilage
18. Thyroid gland
19. Trachea
20. Superior pharyngeal constrictor muscle
21. Middle pharyngeal constrictor muscle
22. Inferior pharyngeal constrictor muscle
23. Esophagus
24. Anterior belly of digastric muscle (cut; innervated by trigeminal nerve)

After Wolf-Heidegger

H&N-60 Oral cavity

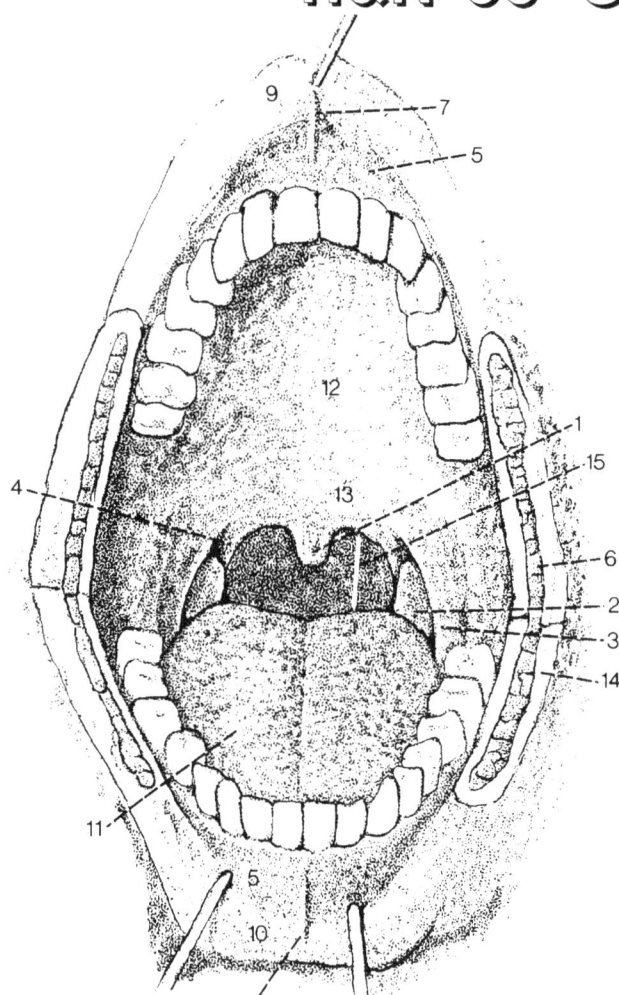

Color and label
1. Uvula (Latin, little grape)
2. Palatine tonsil
3. Palatoglossal arch*
4. Palatopharyngeal arch*
5. Gingiva (Latin, gum)
6. Buccinator muscle (Latin, trumpeter)
7. Frenulum of upper lip (Latin, a small bridle)
8. Frenulum of lower lip
9. Upper lip (Latin, labium superius)
10. Lower lip (Latin, labium inferius)
11. Dorsum of tongue
12. Hard palate
13. Soft palate
14. Cheek (bucca, Latin) (cut)
15. Isthmus of fauces (posterior opening of mouth into pharynx; vertical white line)

*These two arches were also called the pillars of the fauces (Latin, throat).

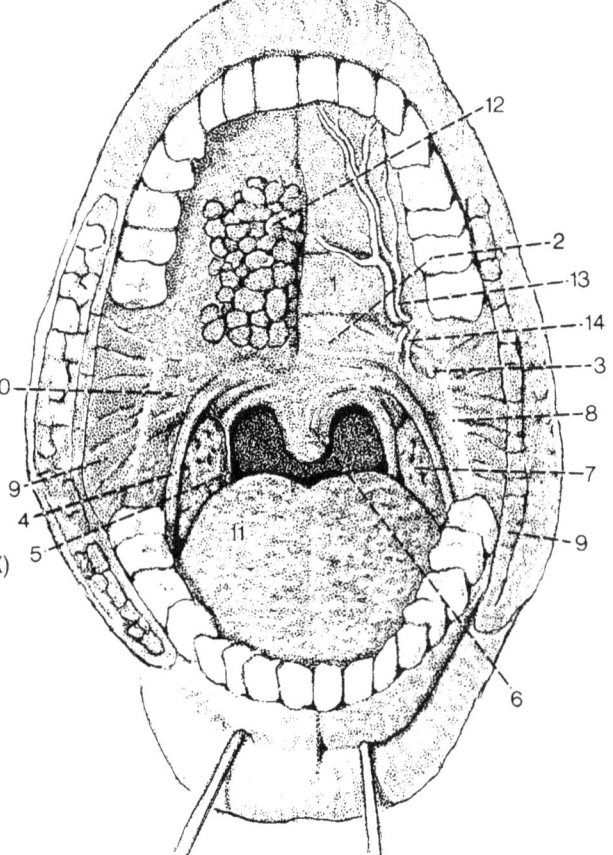

Palatine glands exposed on right side. Glands removed on left side to show greater and lesser palatine nerves.

Color and label
1. Hard palate
2. Soft palate
3. Hamulus (Latin, little hook) of medial pterygoid plate
4. Palatoglossal muscle
5. Palatopharyngeal muscle (both muscles 4 and 5 are innervated by the pharyngeal plexus: nerves IX, X)
6. Muscle of the uvula (musculus uvulae)
7. Palatine tonsil
8. Pterygomandibular raphe (Latin, a seam or suture)
9. Buccinator muscle
10. Superior pharyngeal constrictor muscle
11. Dorsum of tongue
12. Palatine glands
13. Greater palatine vessels and nerve (run forward)
14. Lesser palatine vessels and nerve (run backward)

Redrawn from Spalteholz and Spanner

H&N-60 Oral cavity
(opposite page)

1 _____
2 _____
3 _____
4 _____
5 _____
6 _____
7 _____
8 _____
9 _____
10 _____

11 _____
12 _____
13 _____
14 _____
15 _____

Palatine glands exposed on right side. Glands removed on left side to show greater and lesser palatine nerves.

1 _____
2 _____
3 _____
4 _____
5 _____
6 _____
7 _____
8 _____
9 _____
10 _____

11 _____
12 _____
13 _____
14 _____

H&N-61 Tongue

Inferior surface of tongue and related structures

Color and label
1. Frenulum of tongue
2. Plica fimbriata (Latin, fimbriated fold)
3. Sublingual fold (plica subligualis) (contains openings of sublingual gland ducts)
4. Sublingual caruncle (opening of submandibular duct and main sublingual duct)

After Spalteholz and Spanner

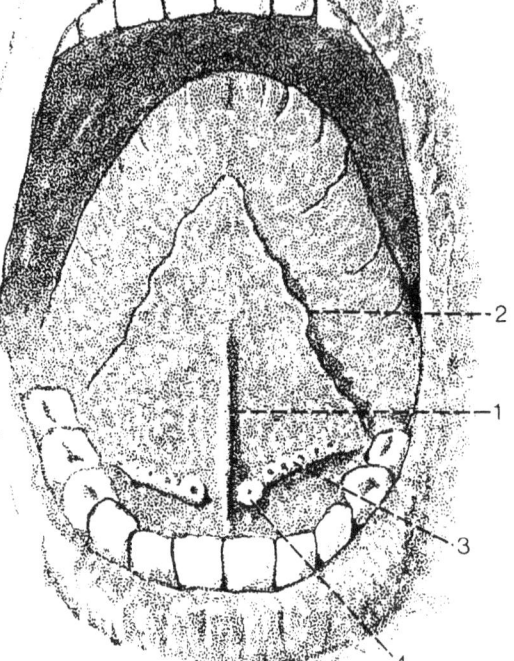

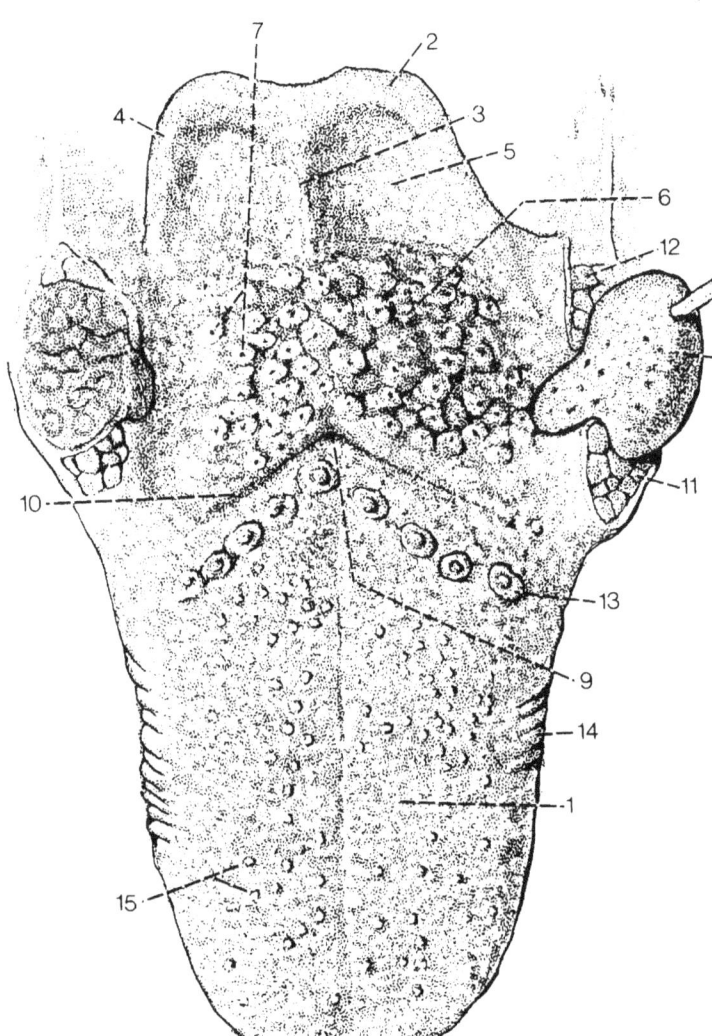

Superior aspect of the tongue and related structures

Color and label
1. Dorsum of tongue
2. Epiglottis
3. Median glosso-epiglottic fold
4. Lateral glosso-epiglottic fold
5. Vallecula (Latin, little valley) epiglottica
6. Lingual tonsil (lymph nodules)
7. Openings of lingual tonsillar crypts
8. Palatine tonsil (often inflamed and removed in childhood)
9. Foramen cecum linguae (blind hole of the tongue)
10. Sulcus terminalis (*sulcus*, akin to the Greek, *holkos*, a furrow)
11. Palatoglossal arch and muscle (cut)
12. Palatopharyngeal arch and muscle (cut)
13. Vallate papilla
14. Foliate papilla (Latin, *folium*, a leaf)
15. Fungiform papilla (Latin, *fungus*, a mushroom)
16. Apex of tongue

After Spalteholz and Spanner

H&N-61 Tongue
(opposite page)

Inferior surface of tongue and related structures

1 _____
2 _____
3 _____
4 _____

Superior aspect of the tongue and related structures

1 _____
2 _____
3 _____
4 _____
5 _____
6 _____
7 _____
8 _____
9 _____
10 _____
11 _____
12 _____
13 _____
14 _____
15 _____
16 _____

H&N-62 Tongue II

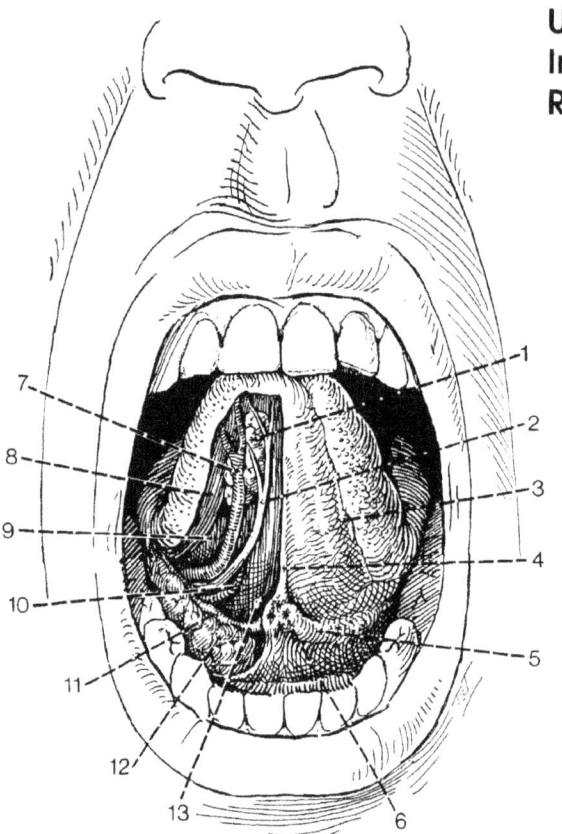

**Upper figure
Inferior surface of tongue
Right side dissected**

Color and label
1. Anterior lingual gland
2. Lingual nerve
3. Fimbriated plica (or fold)
4. Frenulum of tongue
5. Sublingual plica (or fold)
6. Sublingual caruncle
7. Lingual vein
8. Styloglossus muscle
9. Inferior longitudinal muscle of tongue
10. Deep lingual artery
11. Submandibular duct
12. Sublingual gland
13. Genioglossus muscle

**Lower figure
median section of tongue**

Color and label
1. Mandible
2. Hyoid bone
3. Genioglossus muscle
4. Mylohyoid muscle
5. Geniohyoid muscle
6. Superior longitudinal muscle
7. Transverse lingual muscle
8. Foramen cecum of tongue
9. Lingual tonsil(s)
10. Epiglottis
11. Lower lip
12. Vestibule of larynx
13. Vestibular fold (false vocal cord)
14. Vocal fold (vocal cord, true vocal cord)

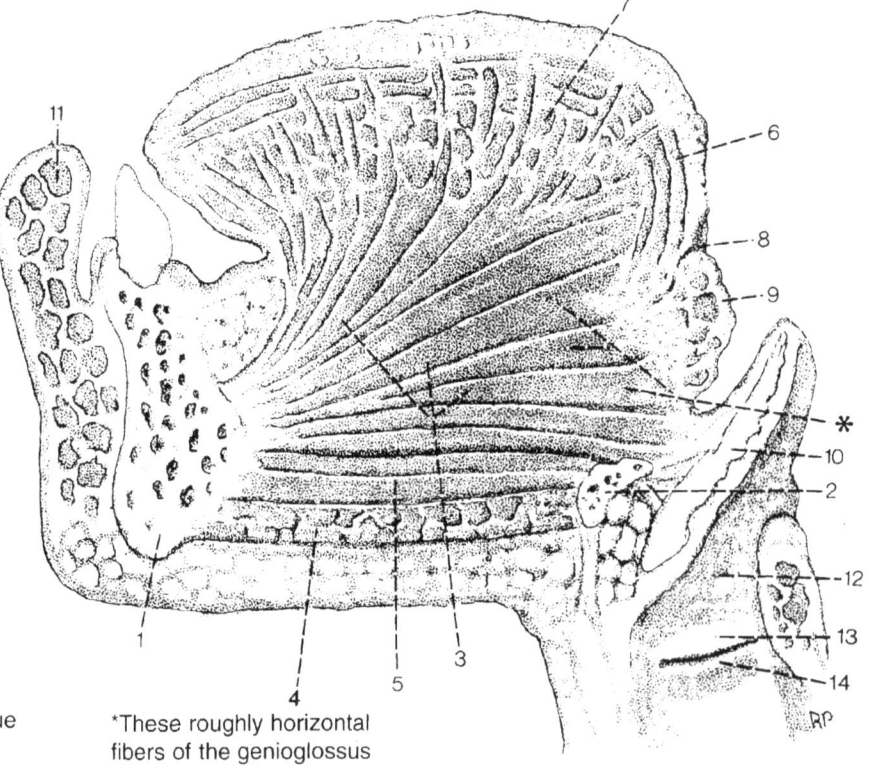

*These roughly horizontal fibers of the genioglossus protrude the tongue.

H&N-62 Tongue II
(opposite page)

Upper figure
Inferior surface of tongue
Right side dissected

1 _____
2 _____
3 _____
4 _____
5 _____
6 _____
7 _____
8 _____
9 _____

10 _____
11 _____
12 _____
13 _____

Lower figure
median section
of tongue

1 _____
2 _____
3 _____
4 _____
5 _____
6 _____
7 _____
8 _____
9 _____

10 _____
11 _____
12 _____
13 _____
14 _____

H&N-63 Tongue and related structures, in coronal section

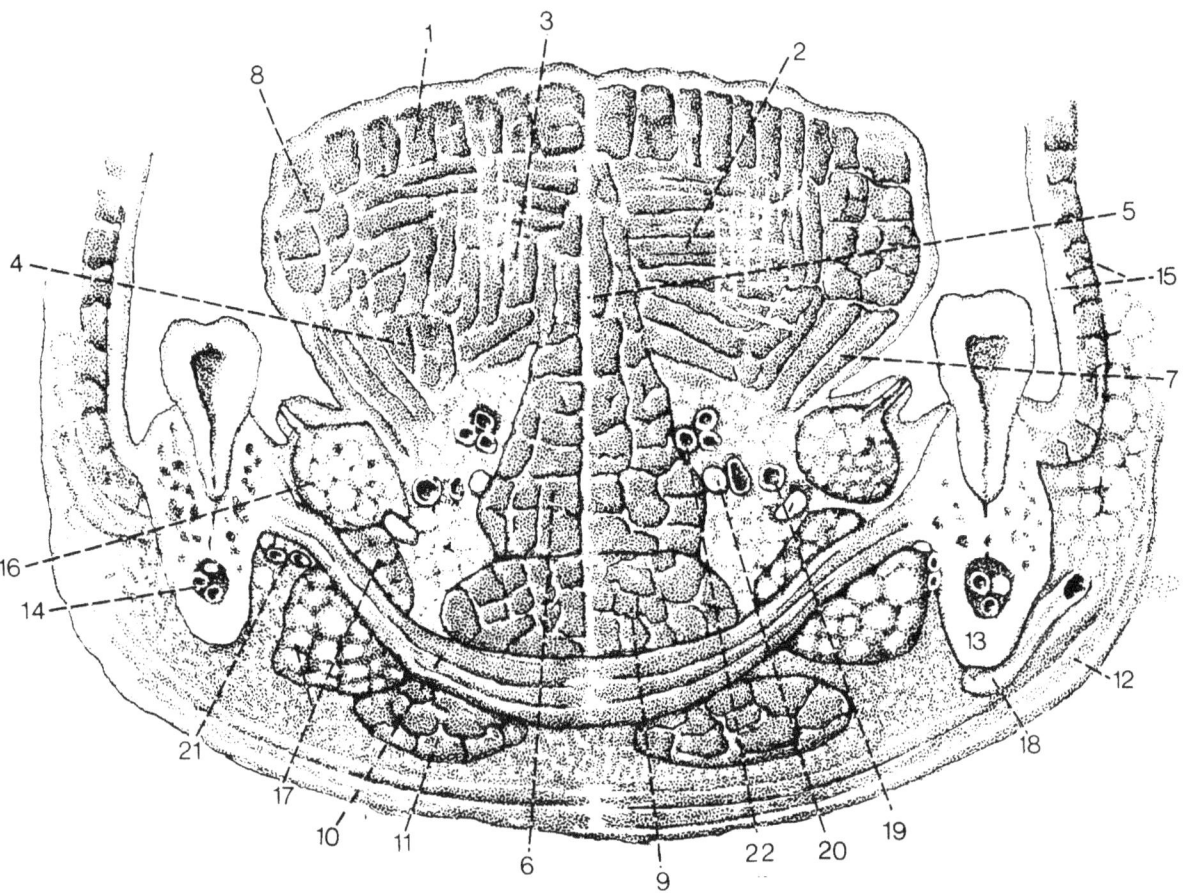

Color and label

1. Superior longitudinal muscle*
2. Transverse lingual muscle*
3. Vertical lingual muscle*
4. Inferior longitudinal muscle*
5. Lingual septum
6. Genioglossus muscle**
7. Hyoglossus muscle**
8. Styloglossus muscle**
9. Geniohyoid muscle
10. Mylohyoid (*myle*, Greek, mill, millstone) muscle
11. Digastric (two-bellied) muscle
12. Platysma muscle
13. Mandible
14. Inferior alveolar nerve, artery, and vein in mandibular canal
15. Buccinator muscle and buccal mucosa (space between tongue and cheek is exaggerated)
16. Sublingual gland and duct opening at sublingual fold
17. Submandibular gland (notice that the gland lies both above and below the mylohyoid muscle)
18. Facial artery
19. Submandibular duct (above) and lingual nerve (below)
20. Hypoglossal nerve and vein
21. Mylohyoid nerve, artery, and vein
22. Deep lingual artery and vein

*Intrinsic muscles of the tongue. They arise and insert within the tongue
**Extrinisic tongue muscles these arise outside the tongue and insert into the tongue.

H&N-63 Tongue and related structures, in coronal section
(opposite page)

1 _____
2 _____
3 _____
4 _____
5 _____
6 _____
7 _____
8 _____
9 _____
10 _____
11 _____

12 _____
13 _____
14 _____
15 _____
16 _____
17 _____
18 _____
19 _____
20 _____
21 _____
22 _____

H&N-64 Temporomandibular joint

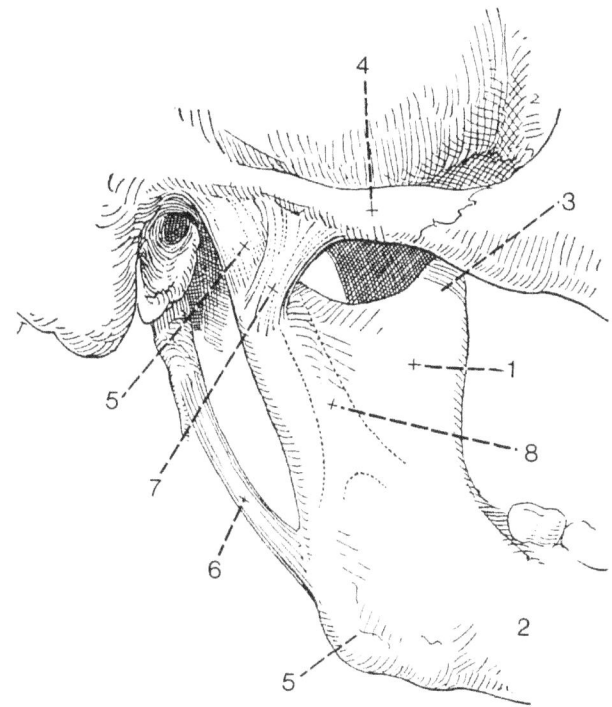

Color and label
1. Ramus of mandible
2. Body of mandible
3. Coronoid process of mandible
4. Zygomatic arch
5. Angle of mandible
6. Stylomandibular ligament
7. Temporomandibular ligament (lateral ligament; medial ligament on inside)
8. Sphenomandibular ligament (on inside of ramus)
9. Head of mandible (partially removed)
10. Articular tubercle
11. Articular disk
12. Mandibular fossa
13. External acoustic meatus
14. Mastoid process
15. Styloid process

Eycleshymer and Jones

**Right temporomandibular joint
Lateral view**

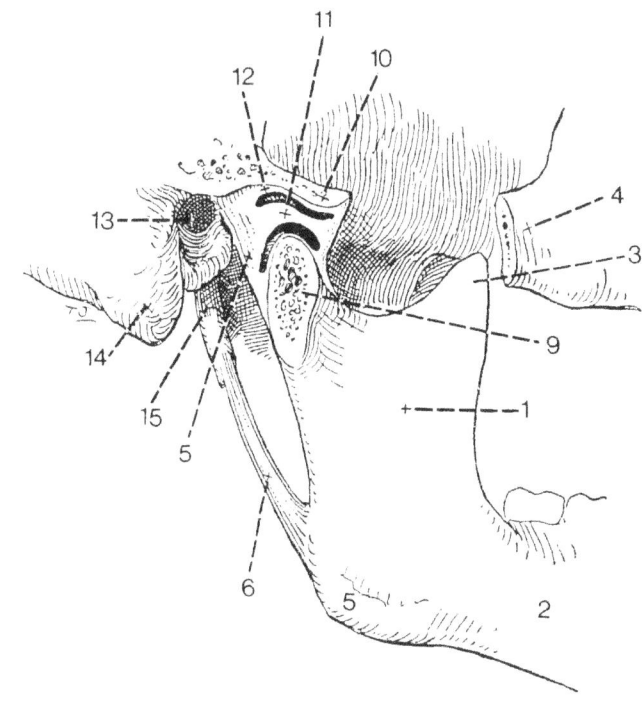

1. _____
2. _____
3. _____
4. _____
5. _____
6. _____
7. _____
8. _____
9. _____
10. _____
11. _____
12. _____
13. _____
14. _____
15. _____

Etymological cartoon: Latin words used to describe parts of the nervous system

1. *Locus ceruleus*, blue place. This mass of nerve cells in the brain derives its name from its blue color.
2. *Tectum*, roof. The former name was *lamina quadrigemina*, the plate with the four bodies–that is, the four colliculi ("little hills").
3. *Vitrum*, glass. *In vitro* means "in glass" (that is, in a test tube or petri dish).
4. *Fenestra*, window. the ear has two small *fenestrae*, the oval window and the round window. Fenestrated capillaries have tiny holes in their walls.
5. *Lithos*, stone (Greek). Otoliths, or ear stones, are found in the inner ear.
6. *Lemniscus*, ribbon. This term describes a flat bundle of axons.
7. *Brachia conjunctiva*, the arms that come together. This was the old name for the superior cerebellar peduncles because the two peduncles would come together and decussate.
8. *Macula*, spot. In ancient Rome instead of calling "here Spot, here Spot" (that is, if you had a dog with a big spot), you would call, "veni macula, veni macula." Immaculate means spotless.
9. *Substantia gelatinosa*, jelly-like substance. This layer of the spinal cord gray matter, now designated layer II of Rexed, appears jelly-like because of the absence of myelinated fibers.
10. *Ampulla*, a swelling or a flask.
11. *Genu*, knee. Geniculate means bent, as in geniculate ganglion or lateral geniculate body. You may wish to genuflect when you encounter an important person, such as an anatomy professor, especially before an exam. You might also wish to address him or her as "your eminence." An eminence is something that rises above its surroundings. In anatomy an eminence means a bump, and in the church or in the palace it was a term of respect for a very important person who rose above his contemporaries.
12. *Peduncle*, little foot or stalk. The cerebellum is attached to the brain stem by six peduncles (three on each side).
13. *Operculum*, a cover or lid. The operculum of the cerebral hemisphere covers the insula.
14. *Amygdala*, almond. This mass of neurons in the temporal lobe has an almond shape.
15. *Putamen*, a shell or husk. This shell-shaped mass of neurons partially envelops the globus pallidus.
16. *Uncus*, hook. The uncinate gyrus on the temporal lobe suggests a hook.
17. *Decussate*, to intersect or to cut in the form of an X.

1. _____
2. _____
3. _____
4. _____
5. _____
6. _____
7. _____
8. _____
9. _____
10. _____
11. _____
12. _____
13. _____
14. _____
15. _____
16. _____
17. _____

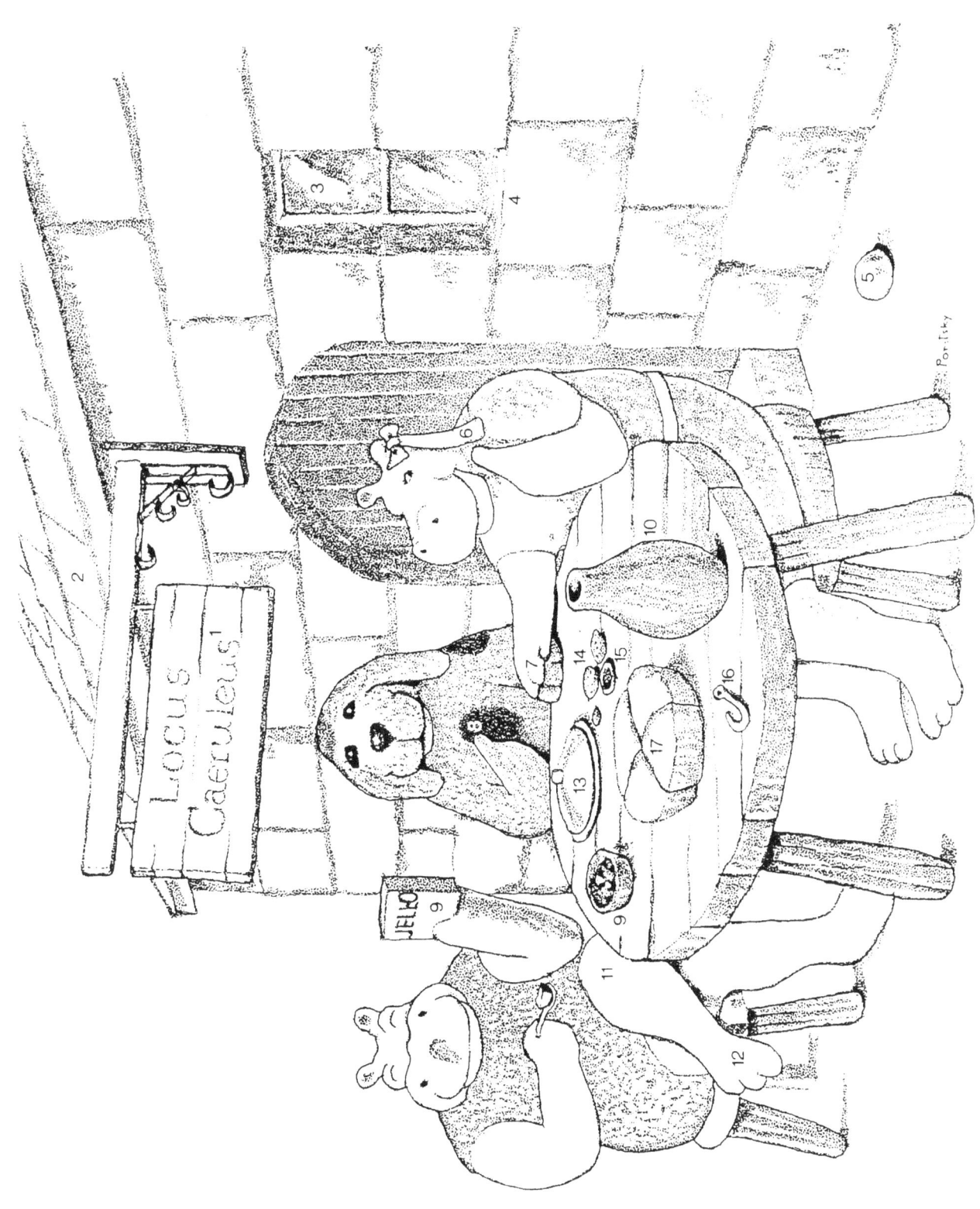

H&N-65 Mandible
(opposite page)

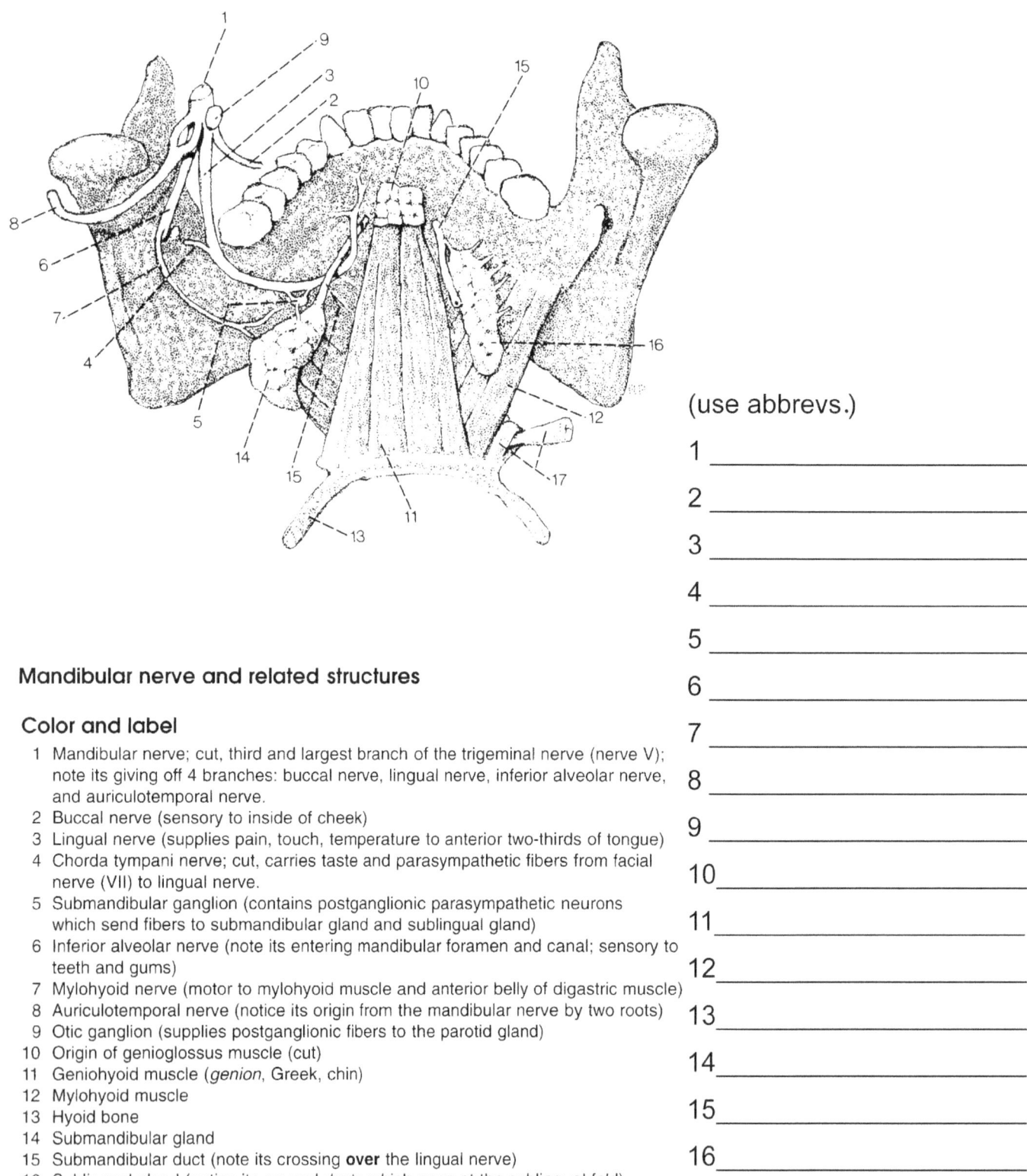

Mandibular nerve and related structures

Color and label

1. Mandibular nerve; cut, third and largest branch of the trigeminal nerve (nerve V); note its giving off 4 branches: buccal nerve, lingual nerve, inferior alveolar nerve, and auriculotemporal nerve.
2. Buccal nerve (sensory to inside of cheek)
3. Lingual nerve (supplies pain, touch, temperature to anterior two-thirds of tongue)
4. Chorda tympani nerve; cut, carries taste and parasympathetic fibers from facial nerve (VII) to lingual nerve.
5. Submandibular ganglion (contains postganglionic parasympathetic neurons which send fibers to submandibular gland and sublingual gland)
6. Inferior alveolar nerve (note its entering mandibular foramen and canal; sensory to teeth and gums)
7. Mylohyoid nerve (motor to mylohyoid muscle and anterior belly of digastric muscle)
8. Auriculotemporal nerve (notice its origin from the mandibular nerve by two roots)
9. Otic ganglion (supplies postganglionic fibers to the parotid gland)
10. Origin of genioglossus muscle (cut)
11. Geniohyoid muscle (*genion*, Greek, chin)
12. Mylohyoid muscle
13. Hyoid bone
14. Submandibular gland
15. Submandibular duct (note its crossing **over** the lingual nerve)
16. Sublingual gland (notice its several ducts which open at the sublingual fold)
17. Digastric muscle posterior belly (cut) and sling restraining intermediate tendon

(use abbrevs.)

1. ___
2. ___
3. ___
4. ___
5. ___
6. ___
7. ___
8. ___
9. ___
10. ___
11. ___
12. ___
13. ___
14. ___
15. ___
16. ___
17. ___

H&N-65 Mandible

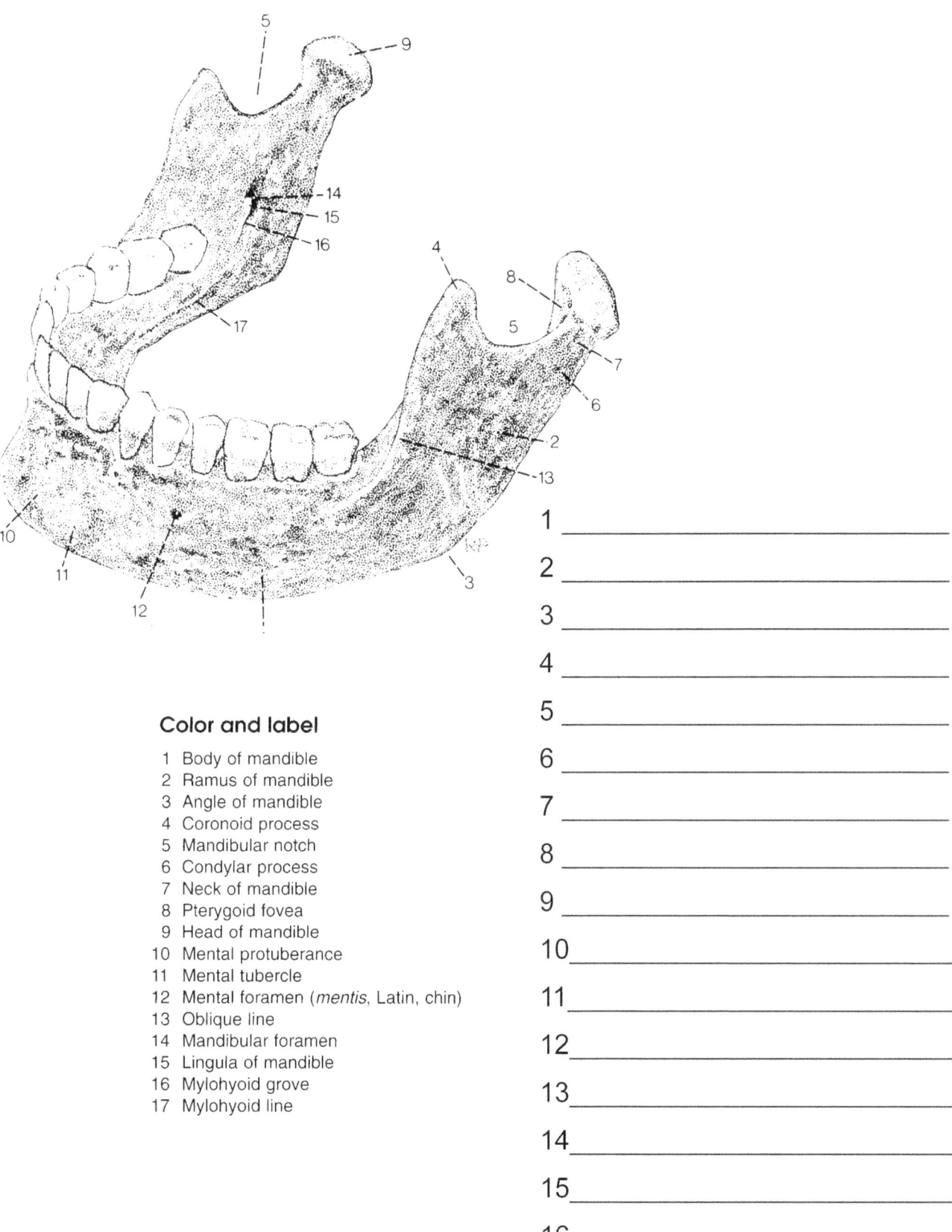

Color and label

1. Body of mandible
2. Ramus of mandible
3. Angle of mandible
4. Coronoid process
5. Mandibular notch
6. Condylar process
7. Neck of mandible
8. Pterygoid fovea
9. Head of mandible
10. Mental protuberance
11. Mental tubercle
12. Mental foramen (*mentis*, Latin, chin)
13. Oblique line
14. Mandibular foramen
15. Lingula of mandible
16. Mylohyoid grove
17. Mylohyoid line

1 _____
2 _____
3 _____
4 _____
5 _____
6 _____
7 _____
8 _____
9 _____
10 _____
11 _____
12 _____
13 _____
14 _____
15 _____
16 _____
17 _____

H&N-66 Salivary glands

Color and label

1. Superficial temporal artery and vein
2. Parotid gland
3. Temporal fascia
4. Buccinator muscle
5. Orbicularis oculi muscle
6. Zygomaticus major muscle
7. Accessory parotid gland
8. Parotid duct
9. Labial glands
10. Gingiva
11. Probe in parotid duct
12. Sublingual caruncle
13. Major sublingual duct
14. Minor sublingual ducts
15. Sublingual gland
16. Lingual nerve
17. Geniohyoid muscle
18. Submandibular duct
19. Hypoglossal nerve
20. Mylohyoid muscle (cut)
21. Hyoglossus muscle
22. Anterior belly of digastric muscle (cut)
23. Submandibular gland
24. Sternohyoid muscle
25. Omohyoid muscle (anterior belly; cut)
26. Sternocleidomastoid muscle
27. Internal jugular vein
28. Greater auricular nerve
29. Posterior belly of digastric muscle
30. Submandibular ganglion
31. Sternocleidomastoid muscle

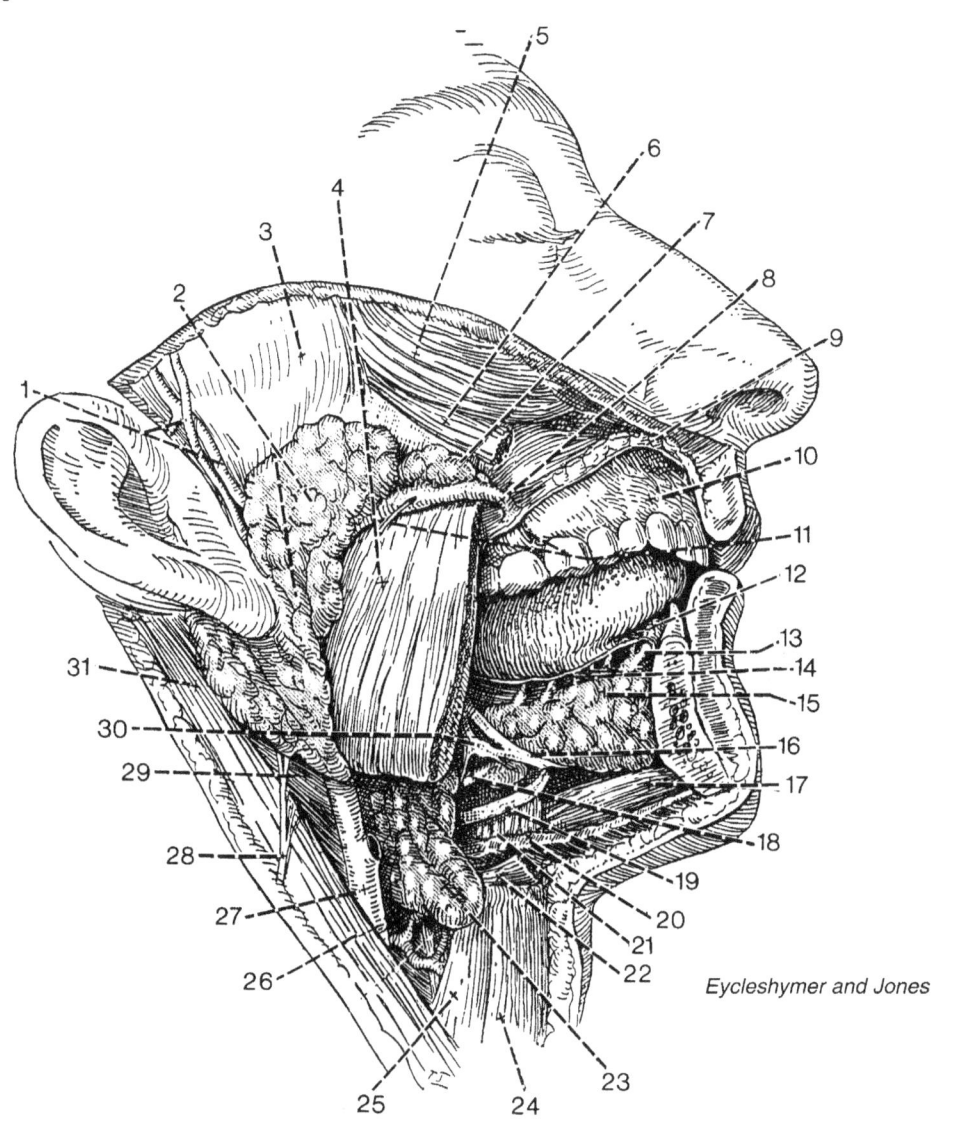

Eycleshymer and Jones

H&N-66 Salivary glands
(opposite page)

1 _____
2 _____
3 _____
4 _____
5 _____
6 _____
7 _____
8 _____
9 _____
10 _____
11 _____
12 _____
13 _____
14 _____
15 _____
16 _____

17 _____
18 _____
19 _____
20 _____
21 _____
22 _____
23 _____
24 _____
25 _____
26 _____
27 _____
28 _____
29 _____
30 _____
31 _____

H&N-67 Oral cavity from inside

Tongue and pharyngeal mucosa and wall removed

Color and label

1. Hard palate
2. Soft palate (cut and removed)
3. Oral mucosa
4. Sublingual papilla
5. Submandibular duct
6. Submandibular gland
7. Sublingual gland and ducts
8. Lingual nerve
9. Hypoglossal nerve (cut)
10. Deep lingual artery (cut)
11. Chorda tympani nerve
12. Inferior alveolar nerve
13. Medial pterygoid muscle (cut)
14. Genioglossus muscle origin on mandible
15. Geniohyoid muscle
16. Mylohyoid muscle
17. Anterior belly of digastric muscle
18. Posterior belly of digastric muscle
19. External carotid artery
20. Internal carotid artery
21. Vagus nerve
22. Ascending pharyngeal artery
23. Facial artery
24. Lingual artery
25. Glossopharyngeal nerve (N IX)
26. Stylohyoid ligament
27. Styloglossus muscle (cut)
28. Hyoglossus muscle (cut)
29. Middle pharyngeal constrictor muscle
30. Hyoid bone
31. Inferior nasal concha

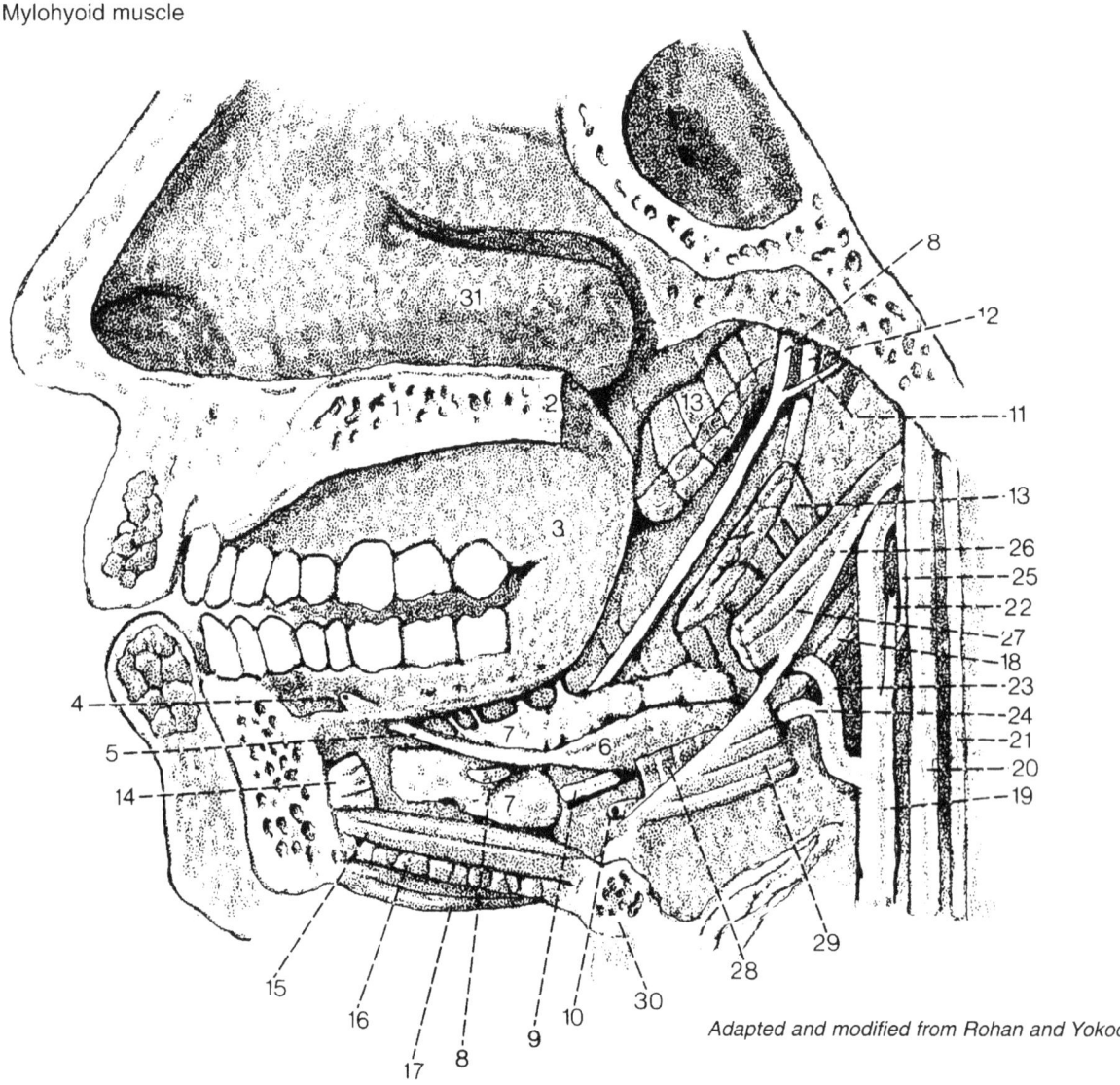

Adapted and modified from Rohan and Yokochi

H&N-67 Oral cavity from inside
Tongue and pharyngeal mucosa and wall removed
(opposite page)

1 _____
2 _____
3 _____
4 _____
5 _____
6 _____
7 _____
8 _____
9 _____
10 _____
11 _____
12 _____
13 _____
14 _____
15 _____
16 _____

17 _____
18 _____
19 _____
20 _____
21 _____
22 _____
23 _____
24 _____
25 _____
26 _____
27 _____
28 _____
29 _____
30 _____
31 _____

H&N-68 Infratemporal fossa

Color and label

1. Facial nerve
2. Retromandibular vein
3. External jugular vein
4. Superficial temporal vein
5. External carotid artery
6. Maxillary artery
7. Superficial temporal vein
8. Middle meningeal artery
9. Masseteric artery
10. Inferior alveolar artery
11. Deep temporal arteries
12. Buccal artery
13. Pterygoid branch
14. Buccal nerve
15. Inferior alveolar nerve
16. Lingual nerve
17. Sphenomandibular ligament
18. Auriculotemporal nerve
19. Facial nerve
20. Ramus of mandible (cut)
21. Neck of mandible (cut)
22. External pterygoid muscle
23. Medial pterygoid muscle
24. Masseter muscle (cut)
25. Buccinator muscle (partially cut)
26. Sternocleidomastoid muscle

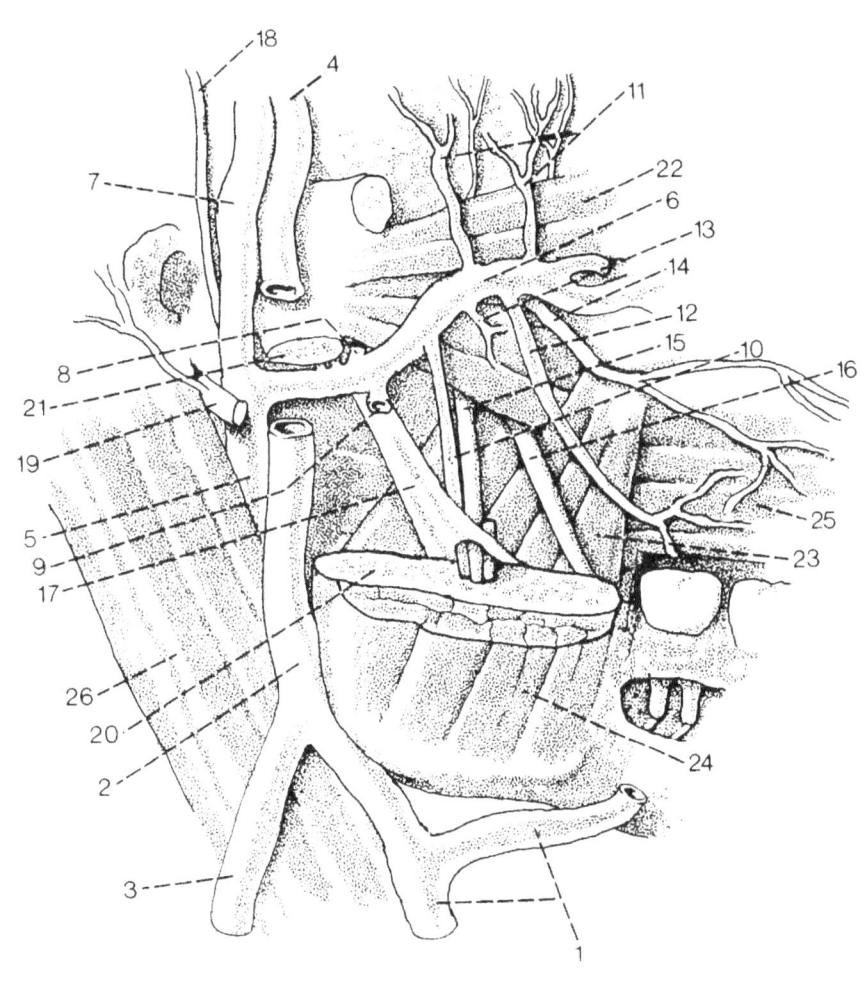

H&N-69 Maxillary artery

(opposite page)

Color and label

1. External carotid artery
2. Maxillary artery
3. Superficial temporal artery
4. Masseteric artery (to masseter muscle)
5. Inferior alveolar artery (supplies teeth in lower jaw; with inferior alveolar vein and nerve; both not shown)
6. Pterygoid branches (supplies pterygoid muscles)
7. Buccal artery (supplies buccinator and cheek)
8. Anterior deep temporal artery (supplies temporalis muscle)
9. Posterior deep temporal artery (supplies temporalis muscle)
10. Posterior superior alveolar artery (supplies upper back teeth)
11. Infraorbital artery (entering orbit)
12. Sphenopalatine artery (entering nose through sphenopalatine foramen)
13. Descending palatine artery
14. Deep auricular artery
15. Anterior tympanic artery
16. Mental artery
17. Lateral pterygoid muscle (superior superficial head)
18. Lateral pterygoid muscle (inferior deep head)
19. Medial pterygoid muscle (superficial head)
20. Medial pterygoid muscle (deep head)
21. Buccinator muscle
22. Masseter muscle (cut)
23. Zygomatic arch (cut)
24. External auditory meatus
25. Temporomandibular joint capsule
26. Ramus of mandible (partially cut, with coronoid process removed)
27. Middle meningeal artery
28. Sternocleidomastoid muscle

Keep in mind: veins, not shown here, travel with arteries and are often doubled; that is, two veins often accompany a single artery.

1 _____
2 _____
3 _____
4 _____
5 _____
6 _____
7 _____
8 _____
9 _____
10 _____
11 _____
12 _____
13 _____
14 _____
15 _____
16 _____
17 _____
18 _____
19 _____
20 _____
21 _____
22 _____
23 _____
24 _____
25 _____
26 _____
27 _____
28 _____

H&N-69 Maxillary artery

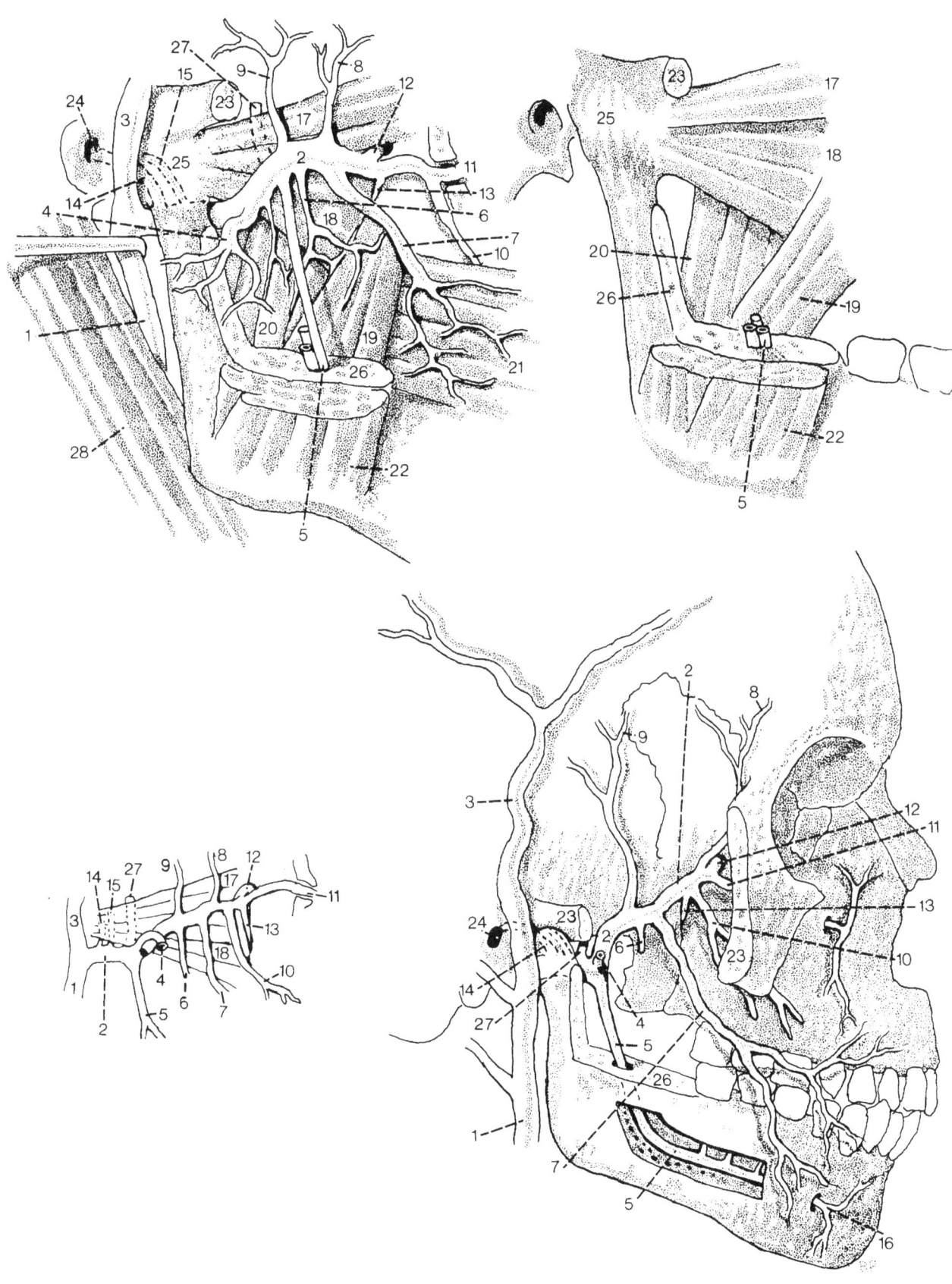

H&N-70 Muscles of the pharynx

Right side (opposite page)

Color and label

1. Auditory tube (cartilaginous)
2. Tensor veli palatini muscle
3. Levator veli palatini muscle
4. Tendon of tensor veli palatini and palatine aponeurosis
5. Hamulus of medial pterygoid plate
6. Pterygomandibular raphe
7. Buccinator muscle
8. Superior pharyngeal constrictor muscle
9. Palatopharyngeus muscle
10. Salpingopharyngeus muscle
11. Glossopharyngeus muscle (part of superior constrictor)
12. Middle pharyngeal constrictor muscle
13. Styloglossus muscle
14. Hyoglossus muscle
15. Stylohyoid ligament
16. Inferior pharyngeal constrictor muscle
17. Mylohyoid muscle
18. Geniohyoid muscle
19. Thyrohyoid membrane
20. Stylopharyngeus muscle
21. Fibers to pharyngo-epiglottic fold
22. Longitudinal muscle of pharynx
23. Internal branch of superior laryngeal nerve
24. Thyroid cartilage
25. Cricoid cartilage
26. Trachea
27. Arytenoid cartilage
28. Corniculate cartilage
29. Pharyngeal aponeurosis
30. Cricopharyngeus muscle (part of inferior constrictor)
31. Esophageal circular muscle
32. Esophageal longitudinal muscle
33. Pharyngobasilar fascia
34. Hyoid bone

H&N-70 Muscles of the pharynx

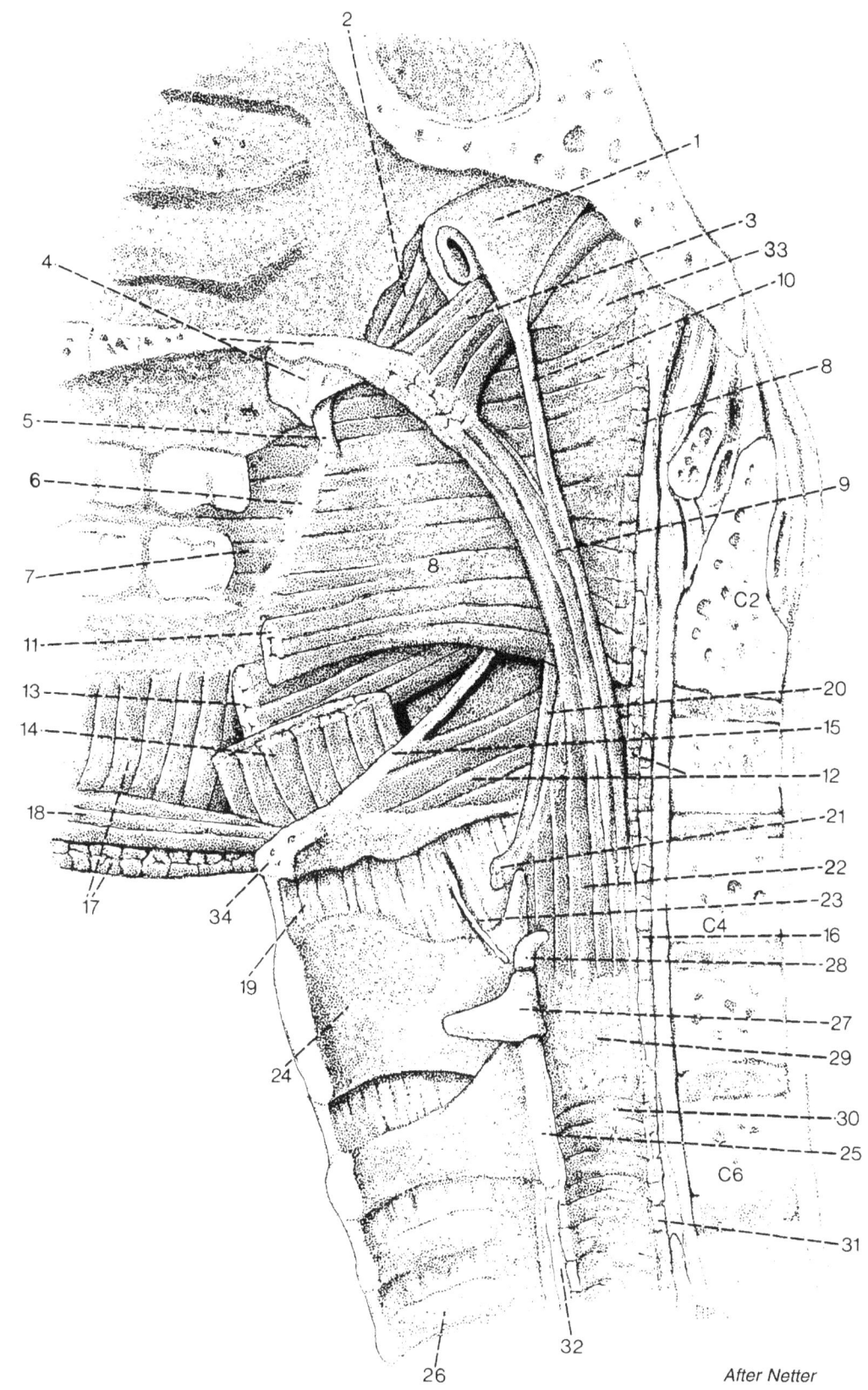

After Netter

H&N-71 Arytenoid and cricoid cartilages

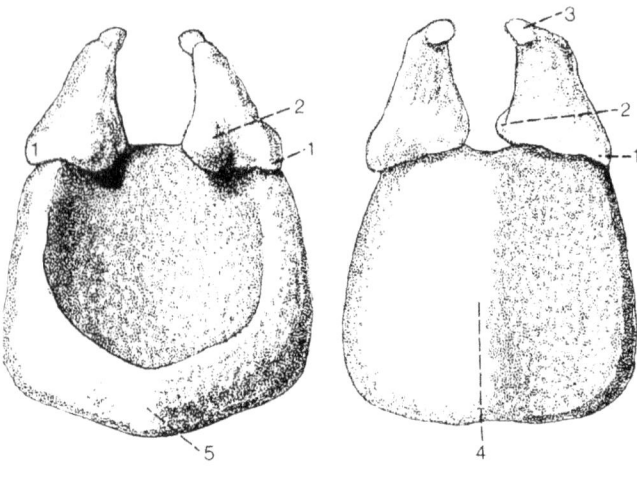

Anterior   Posterior

**Left, anterior view;
Right, posterior view**

Color and label
1 Muscular process of arytenoid cartilage
2 Vocal process of arytenoid cartilage
3 Corniculate cartilage
4 Lamina of cricoid cartilage
5 Arch of cricoid cartilage

1 _____
2 _____
3 _____
4 _____
5 _____

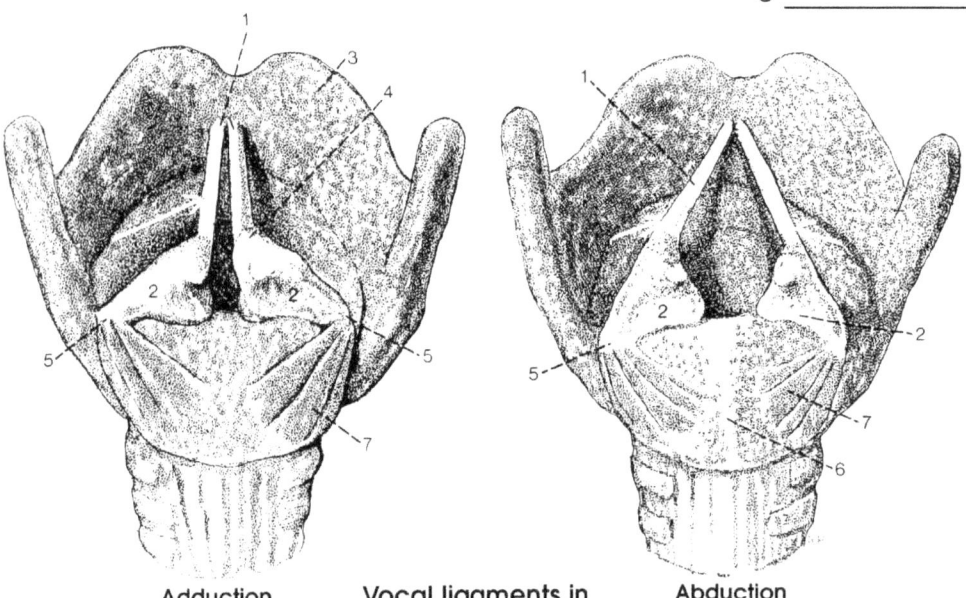

Adduction   Vocal ligaments in   Abduction

Color and label
1 Vocal ligaments
2 Arytenoid cartilages
3 Thyroid cartilage
4 Vocal process of arytenoid cartilage
5 Muscular process of arytenoid cartilage
6 Lamina of cricoid cartilage
7 Posterior cricoarytenoid muscles; these two muscles are the sole abductors (pull apart) of the vocal ligaments, thus opening the space between the vocal cords (the rima glottidis).
8 White arrows indicate the conus elasticus (not shown here, see next page); these extend from the cricoid cartilage to the vocal ligaments.

1 _____
2 _____
3 _____
4 _____
5 _____
6 _____
7 _____
8 _____

H&N-72 Vocal ligaments and muscles

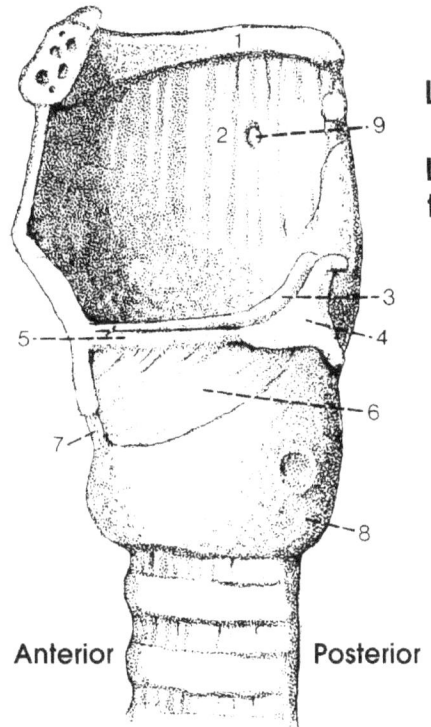

Larynx partially bisected

Left half of hyoid bone and thryroid cartilage removed

Color and label

1. Right half of hyoid bone
2. Right thyrohyoid membrane
3. Right arytenoid cartilage
4. Left arytenoid cartilage
5. Vocal ligaments
6. Conus elasticus
7. Cricothyroid ligament
8. Cricoid cartilage
9. Foramen for passage of internal branch of superior laryngeal nerve and artery

1 _____
2 _____
3 _____
4 _____
5 _____
6 _____
7 _____
8 _____
9 _____

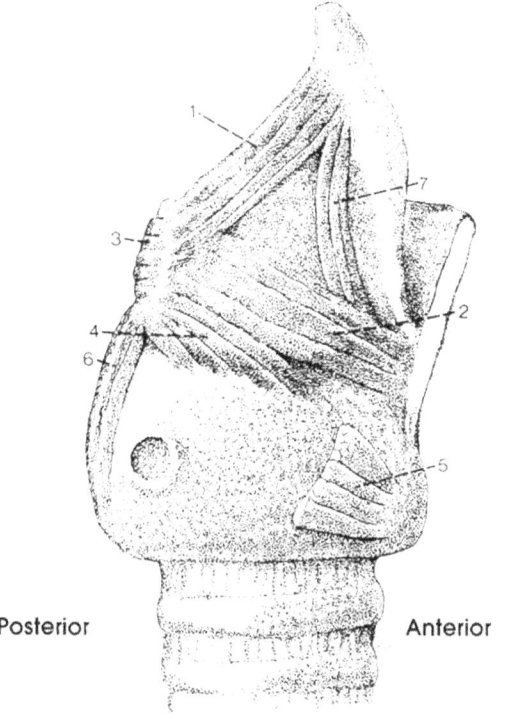

Muscles of right side of larynx

Right side of thyroid cartilage removed

Color and label

1. Aryepiglottis muscle
2. Thyroarytenoid muscle
3. Arytenoid muscle muscle
4. Lateral cricoarytenoid muscle
5. Cricothyroid muscle
6. Posterior cricoarytenoid muscle

1 _____
2 _____
3 _____
4 _____
5 _____
6 _____

H&N-73 Larynx, cartilages

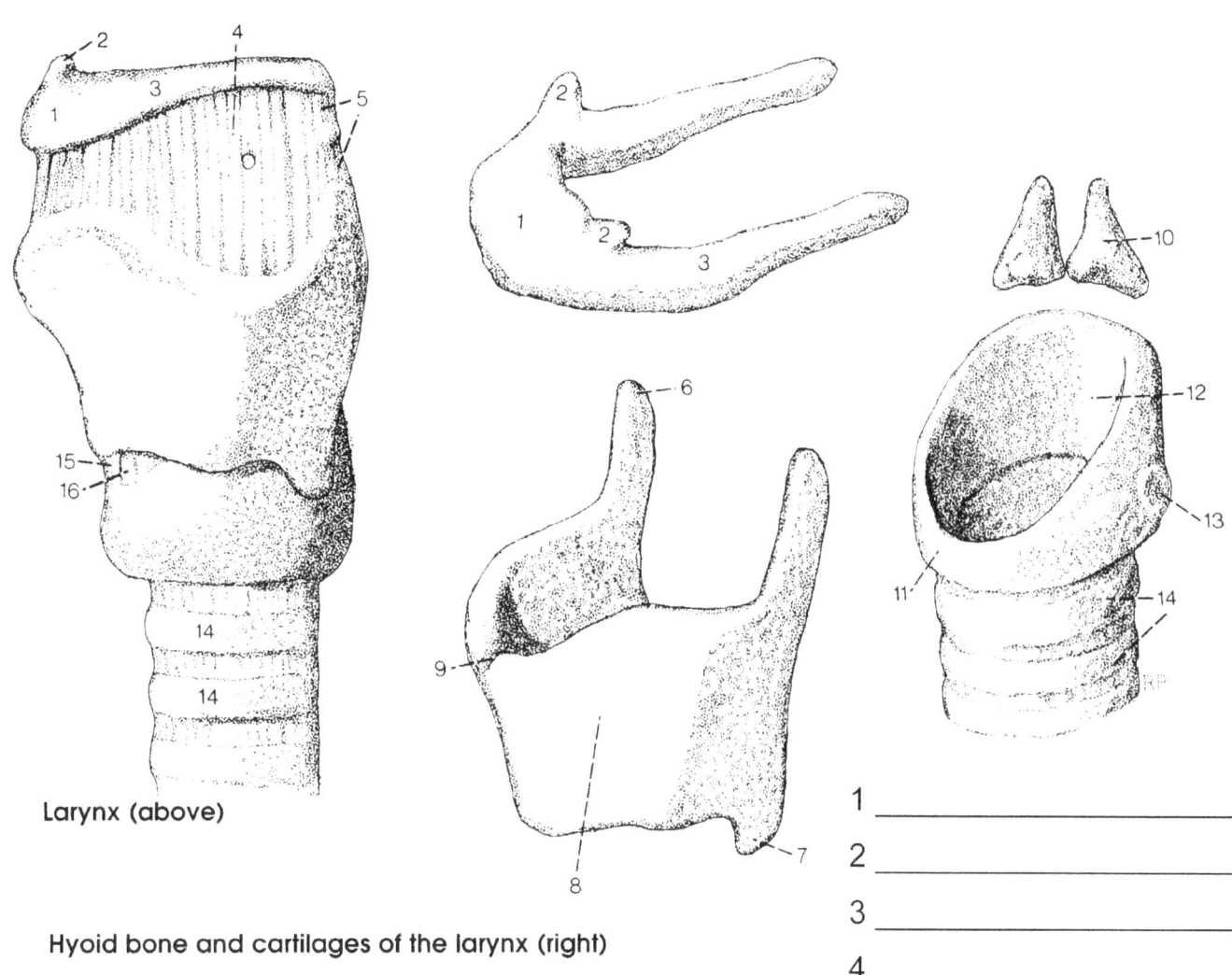

Larynx (above)

Hyoid bone and cartilages of the larynx (right)

Color and label

1. Body of hyoid bone
2. Lesser horn (cornu) of hyoid bone
3. Greater horn (cornu) of hyoid bone
4. Thyrohyoid membrane
5. Lateral thyrohyoid ligament
6. Superior horn of thyroid cartilage
7. Inferior horn of thyroid cartilage
8. Lamina of thyroid cartilage
9. Superior thyroid notch
10. Arytenoid (Greek, *arytaina*, pitcher, ladle) cartilage
11. Arch of cricoid cartilage
12. Lamina of cricoid cartilage
13. Facet for inferior horn of thyroid cartilage
14. Tracheal rings
15. Cricothyroid ligament
16. Conus elasticus (extends from cricoid cartilage to vocal ligament

1 _____
2 _____
3 _____
4 _____
5 _____
6 _____
7 _____
8 _____
9 _____
10 _____
11 _____
12 _____
13 _____
14 _____
15 _____
16 _____

H&N-74 Pharynx

Posterior aspect (opposite page)

Color and label

1. Nasal septum
2. Nasal conchae
3. Pharyngeal
4. Pharyngeal wall (cut open along posterior raphe)
5. Nasal pharynx (nasopharynx)
6. Oral pharynx (oropharynx)
7. Laryngeal pharynx (laryngopharynx)
8. Soft palate and uvula
9. Dorsum sellae and clivus (Latin, slope) of occipital bone
10. Petrous portion of temporal bone
11. Facial canal and its termination at the stylomastoid foramen
12. Styloid process
13. Mastoid process and mastoid air cells
14. Opening of auditory tube
15. Torus tubularis
16. Torus of levator veli palatini muscle
17. Pharyngeal recess
18. Palatopharyngeal fold
19. Palatine tonsil
20. Root of tongue (posterior third) with lingual lymph follicles (tonsil)
21. Epiglottis
22. Piriform recess
23. Superior laryngeal nerve and vessel under mucous membrane
24. Hyoid bone (greater horn)
25. Thyroid cartilage (superior horn)
26. Interarytenoid notch
27. Corniculate tubercle (covering corniculate cartilage)
28. Cuneiform tubercle (covering cuneiform cartilage)
29. Aryepiglottic fold
30. Esophagus
31. Thyroid gland and vessels
32. Parathyroid gland
33. Mucous membrane overlying posterior cricoarytenoid and lamina of cricoid cartilage
34. Aditus (Latin, entrance) to larynx
35. Vallate papillae
36. Posterior belly of digastric muscle
37. Parotid gland
38. Submandibular gland

1 _____
2 _____
3 _____
4 _____
5 _____
6 _____
7 _____
8 _____
9 _____
10 _____
11 _____
12 _____
13 _____
14 _____
15 _____
16 _____
17 _____
18 _____
19 _____
20 _____
21 _____
22 _____
23 _____
24 _____
25 _____
26 _____
27 _____
28 _____
29 _____
30 _____
31 _____
32 _____
33 _____
34 _____
35 _____
36 _____
37 _____
38 _____

H&N-74 Pharynx

Posterior aspect

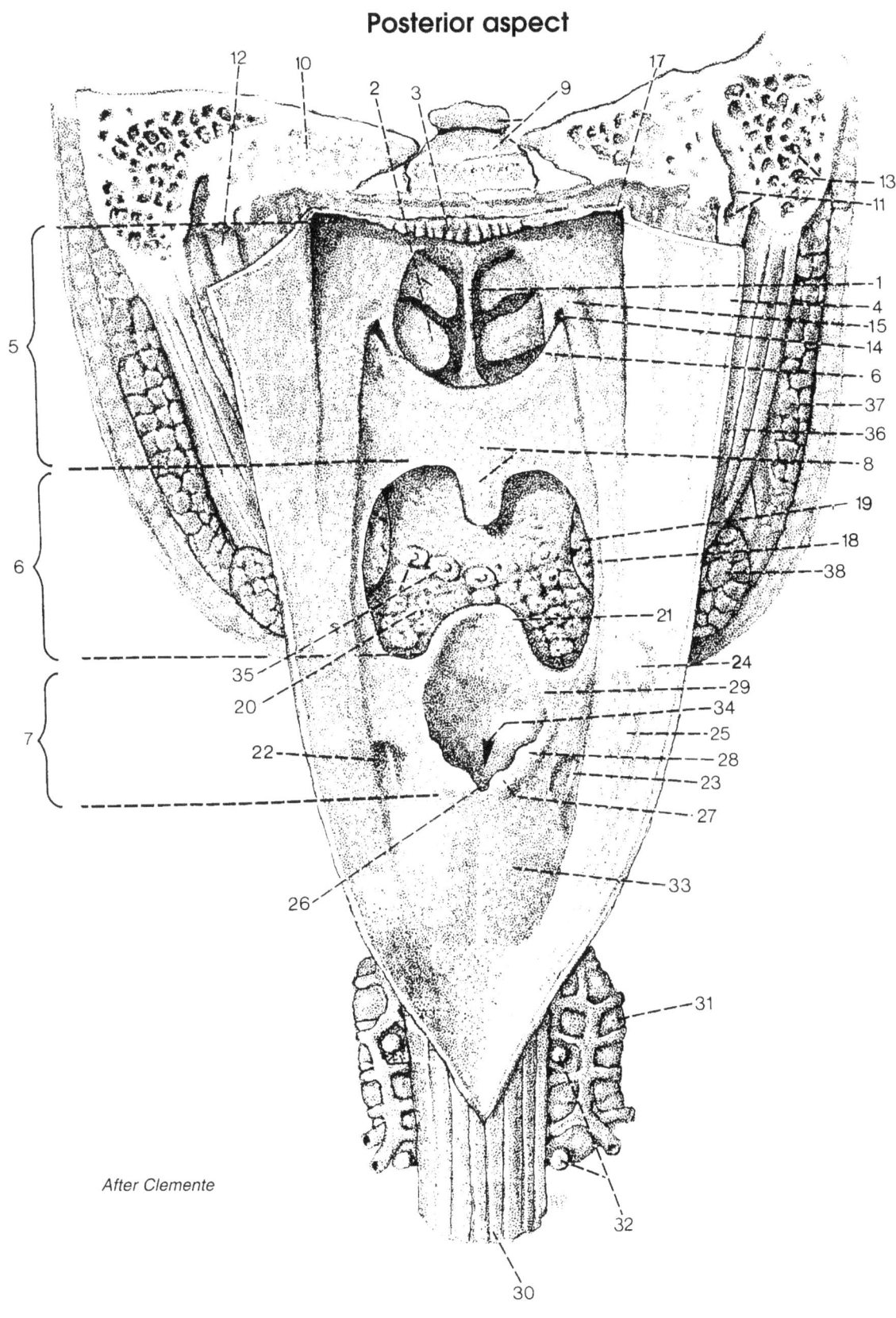

After Clemente

H&N-75 Arytenoid cartilages

Color and label
1. Right arytenoid cartilage (anterolateral aspect)
2. Left arytenoid cartilage
3. Corniculate cartilage
4. Apex of arytenoid cartilage
5. Neck
6. Triangilar fossa
7. Arcuate crest
8. Base of arytenoid cartilage
9. Oblong fossa
10. Muscular process
11. Vocal process
12. Vocal ligaments (cut)
13. Conus elasticus (cut) (cricovocal membrane)
14. Cricoid cartilage (cut)
15. Vestibular ligament (cut)
16. Vocalis muscle (cut)
17. Thyroarytenoid muscle (cut)
18. Lateral cricoarytenoid muscle (cut)

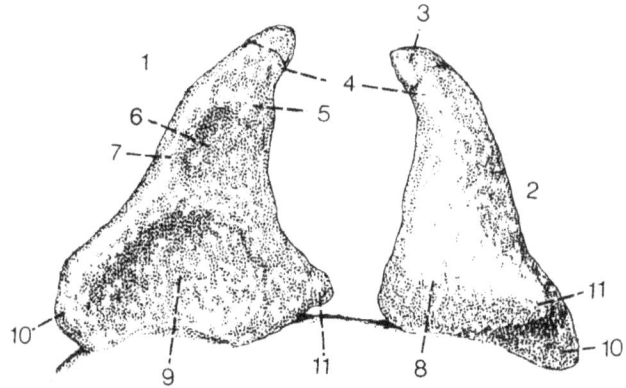
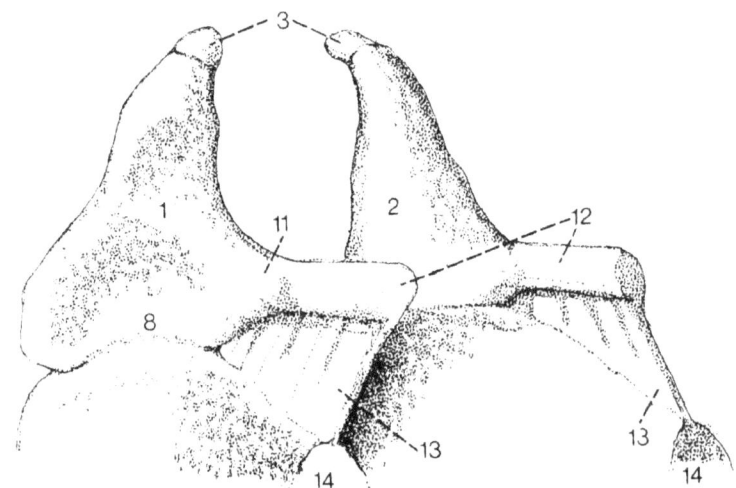
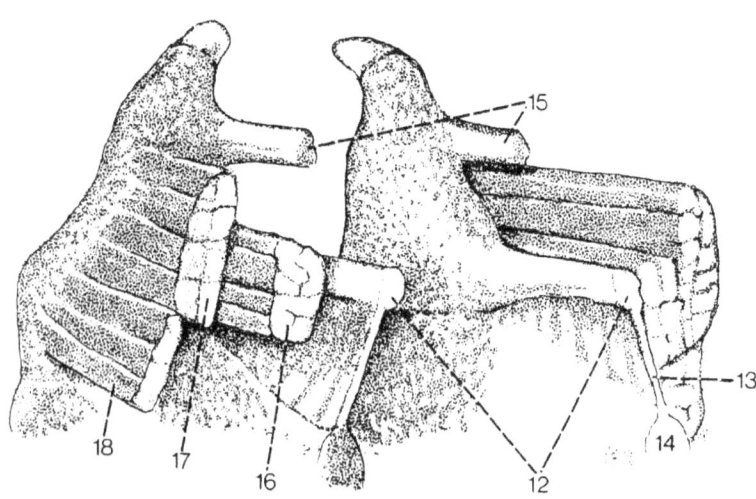

1. _____
2. _____
3. _____
4. _____
5. _____
6. _____
7. _____
8. _____
9. _____
10. _____
11. _____
12. _____
13. _____
14. _____
15. _____
16. _____
17. _____
18. _____

H&N-76 Larynx, cartilages
Posterior aspect

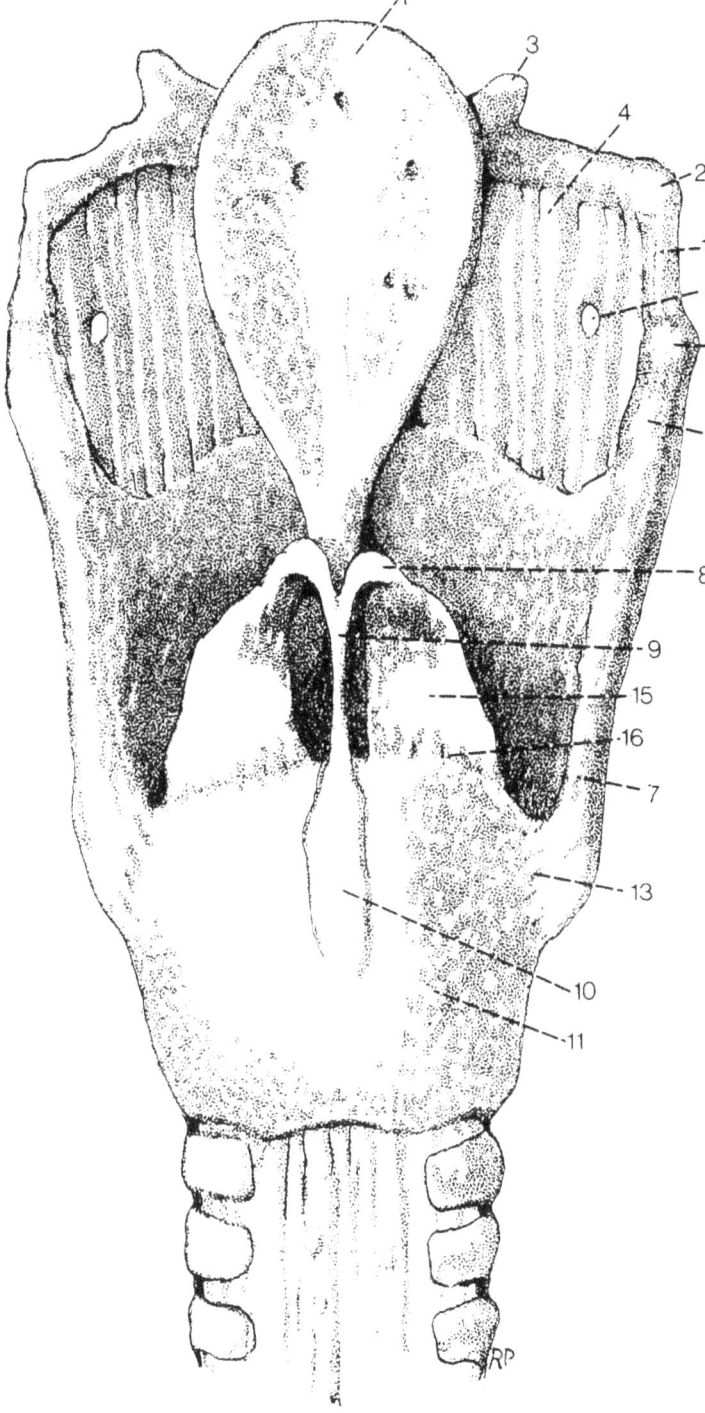

Color and label
1. Epiglottis
2. Hyoid bone greater horn
3. Hyoid bone lesser horn
4. Thyrohyoid membrane
5. Foramen for internal branch of superior laryngeal nerve and superior laryngeal artery
6. Superior horn of thyroid cartilage
7. Inferior horn of thyroid cartilage
8. Corniculate cartilage
9. Corniculopharyngeal ligament
10. Cricopharyngeal ligament
11. Lamina of cricoid cartilage
12. Triticeal cartilage
13. Cricothyroid joint and ligament
14. Lateral thyrohyoid ligament
15. Arytenoid cartilage
16. Cricoarytenoid joint and ligament

1 _____
2 _____
3 _____
4 _____
5 _____
6 _____
7 _____
8 _____
9 _____
10 _____
11 _____
12 _____
13 _____
14 _____
15 _____
16 _____

H&N-77 Larynx, nerves and muscles

Posterior view

Color and label

1. Posterior cricoarytenoid muscle (only abductor of the vocal folds)
2. Oblique arytenoid muscle
3. Transverse arytenoid muscle
4. Aryepiglottic muscle (also considered part of oblique arytenoid)
5. Inferior laryngeal nerve
6. Recurrent laryngeal nerve
7. Membranous tracheal wall and glands
8. Epiglottis
9. Interarytenoid notch
10. Cuneiform cartilage and tubercle
11. Internal branch of superior laryngeal nerve
12. Superior laryngeal artery

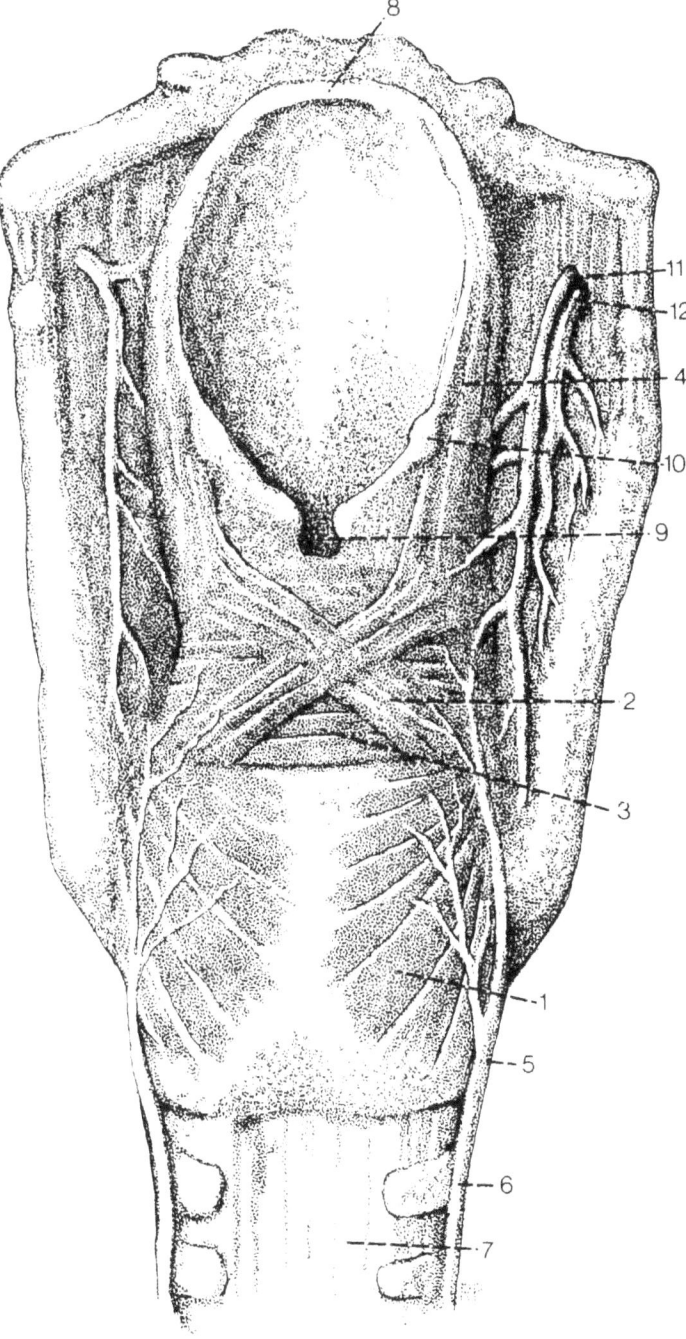

1 _____
2 _____
3 _____
4 _____
5 _____
6 _____
7 _____
8 _____
9 _____
10 _____
11 _____
12 _____

H&N-78 Larynx, coronal section

Viewed from behind

Figure A and B (opposite page)

Color and label

1. Vestibular fold (false vocal cord)
2. Vestibular ligament
3. Ventricle of larynx
4. Vocal ligament
5. Vocal fold (true vocal cord)
6. Vocalis muscle
7. Thyroarytenoid muscle
8. Lateral cricoarytenoid muscle
9. Rima glottidis (space between vocal folds); divided into: intermembranous part, intercartilaginous part, interarytenoid fold
10. Cricothyroid muscle
11. Arch of cricoid cartilage
12. Tracheal rings
13. Epiglottis
14. Vestibule of larynx (laryngeal space above vestibular folds)
15. Infraglottic space (laryngeal space below vocal folds)
16. Hyoid bone
17. Conus elasticus (cricovocal membrane)
18. Aryepiglottic muscle
19. Thyrohyoid muscle
20. Rima glottidis (intermembranous part)
21. Rima glottidis (intercartilaginous part)
22. Root of tongue (posterior one-third)
23. Palatine tonsil
24. Piriform recess
25. Cuneiform tubercle
26. Corniculate tubercle
27. Interarytenoid notch
28. Laryngeal pharynx leading to esophagus
29. Epiglottic depression (vallecula epiglottica)
30. Aryepiglottic fold

1. _____
2. _____
3. _____
4. _____
5. _____
6. _____
7. _____
8. _____
9. _____
10. _____
11. _____
12. _____
13. _____
14. _____
15. _____
16. _____
17. _____
18. _____
19. _____
20. _____
21. _____
22. _____
23. _____
24. _____
25. _____
26. _____
27. _____
28. _____
29. _____
30. _____

H&N-78 Larynx, coronal section
Larynx and surrounding structures

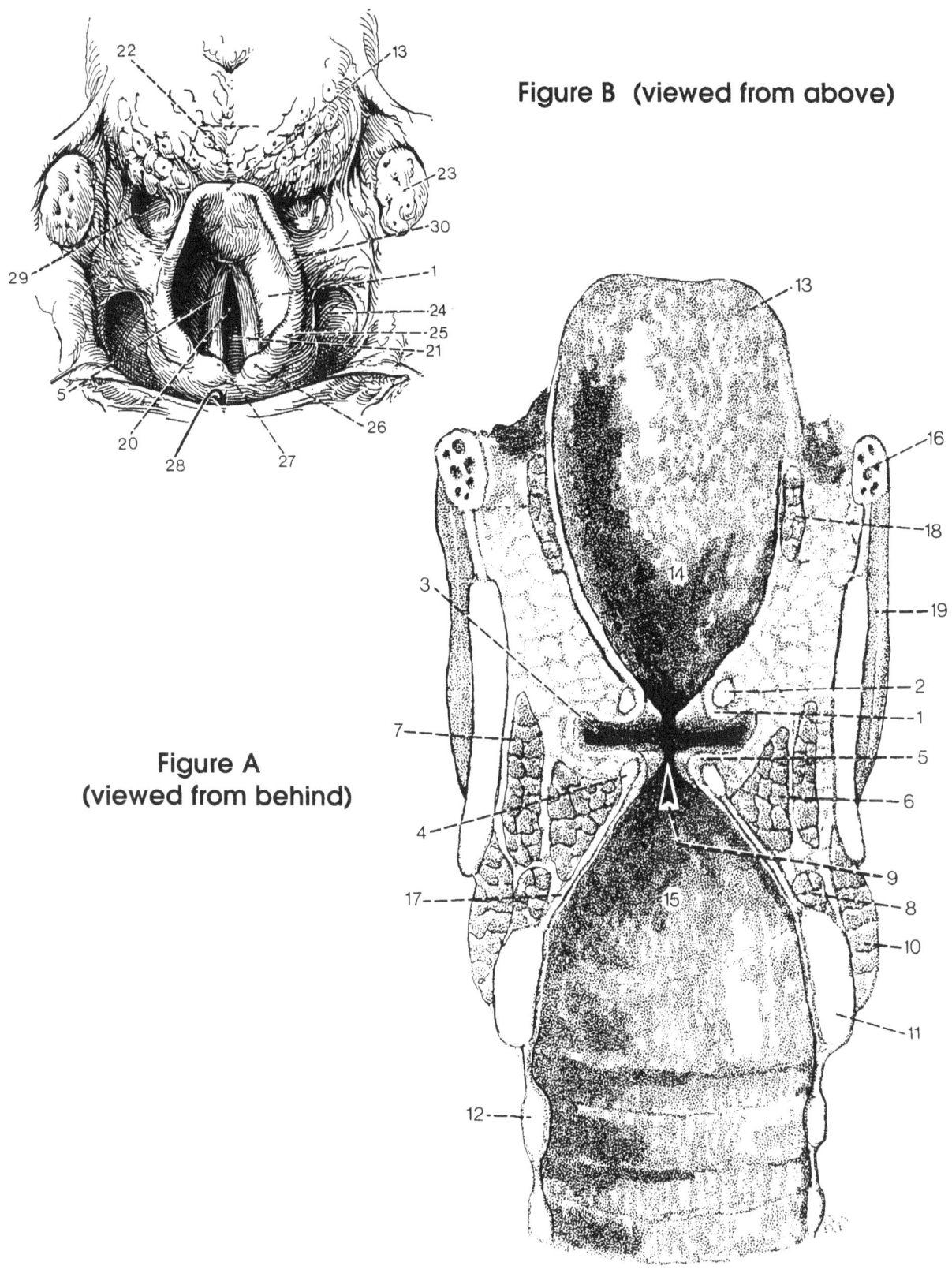

Figure B (viewed from above)

Figure A (viewed from behind)

H&N-79 Muscle origins and insertions on side of skull

Color the origins (O) RED and the insertions (I) BLUE

1. Temporalis (O)
2. Temporalis (I)
3. Masseter (O)
4. Masseter (I)
5. Buccinator (O)*
6. Zygomatic major (O)
7. Orbicularis oculi (orbital part) (O)
8. Corrugator supercilii (O)
9. Orbicularis oculi (lacrimal part) (O)
10. Levator labii superioris alaeque nasi (O)
11. Orbicularis oculi (orbital part) (O)
12. Zygomatic minor (O)
13. Levator labii superioris (O)
14. Compressor naris (O)
15. Levator anguli oris (O)
16. Orbicularis oris (O)
17. Mentalis (O)
18. Orbicularis oris (O)
19. Depressor labii inferioris (O)
20. Depressor anguli oris (O)
21. Sternocleidomastoid (I)
22. Occipitalis (O)
23. Trapezius (O)
24. Semispinalis capitis (I)
25. Obliquus capitis superior (I)
26. Rectus capitis posterior major (I)
27. Rectus capitis posterior minor (I)
28. Splenius capitis (I)
29. Digastric (O)
30. Longissimus capitis (I)
31. Stylohyoid (O)
32. Styloglossus (O)
33. Platysma (O)

*The muscles of facial expression insert mainly on the deep skin rather than on bone.

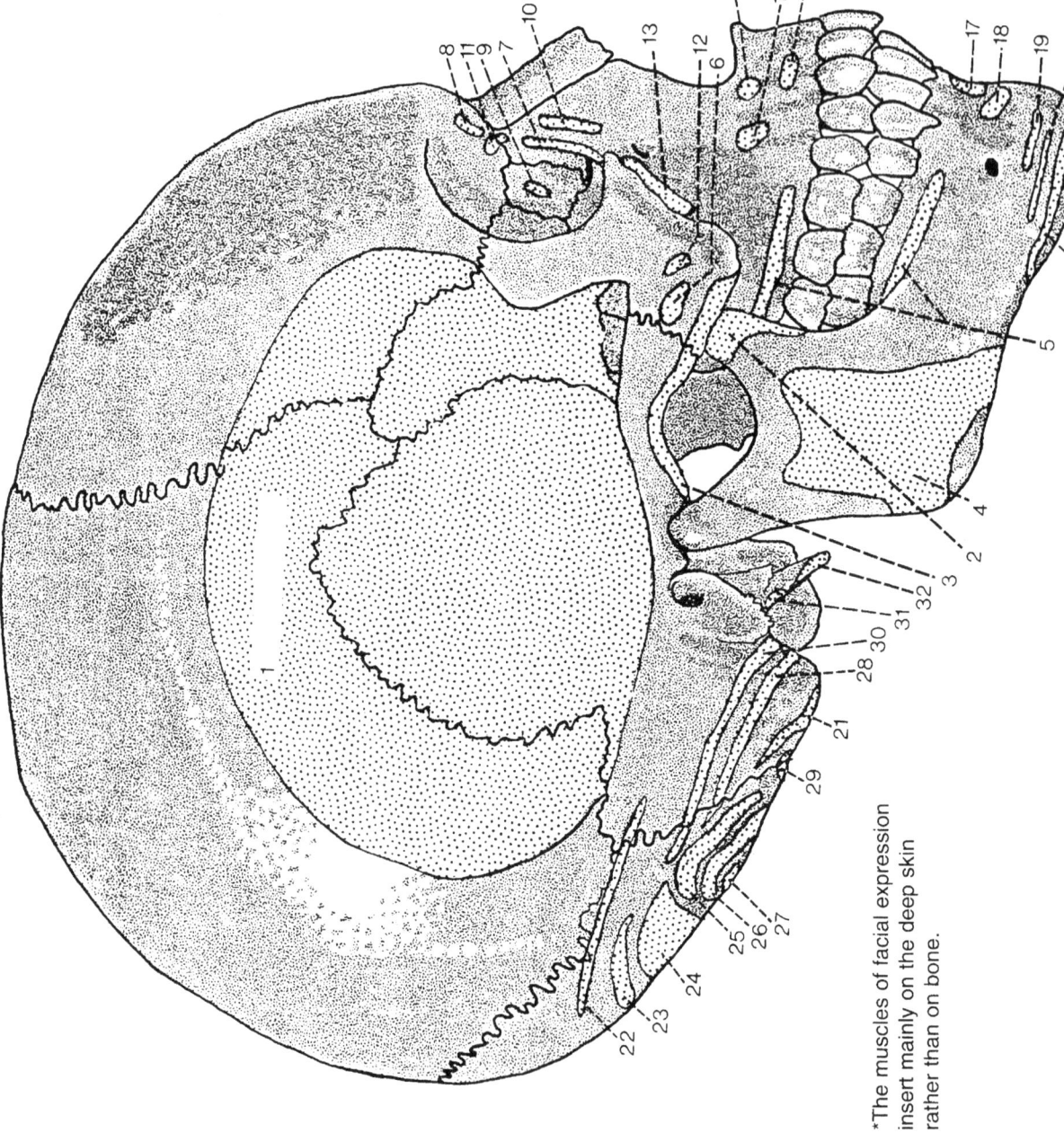

H&N-79 Muscle origins and insertions on side of skull
(opposite page)

1 _____
2 _____
3 _____
4 _____
5 _____
6 _____
7 _____
8 _____
9 _____
10 _____
11 _____
12 _____
13 _____
14 _____
15 _____
16 _____
17 _____

18 _____
19 _____
20 _____
21 _____
22 _____
23 _____
24 _____
25 _____
26 _____
27 _____
28 _____
29 _____
30 _____
31 _____
32 _____
33 _____

H&N-80 Skull

Inferior aspect

Color each bone a different color

Temporal (T)
Sphenoid (S)
Occipital (O)
Zygomatic (Z)
Maxillary (M)
Palatine (Pal)
Vomer (V)

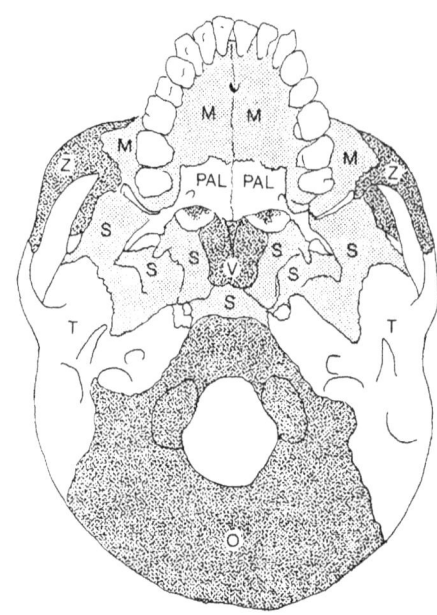

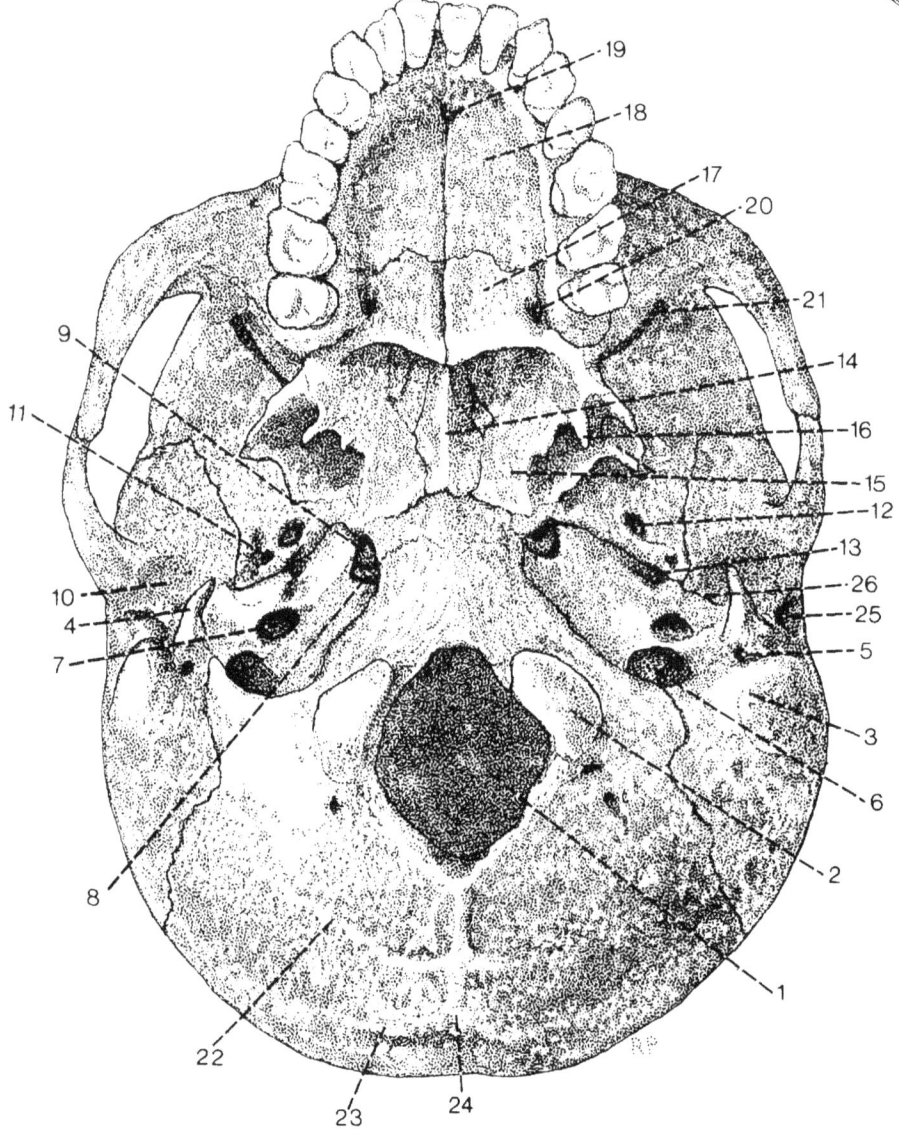

...and label

1. Foramen magnum
2. Occipital condyle
3. Mastoid foramen
4. Styloid process
5. Stylomastoid foramen
6. Jugular foramen
7. Carotid canal external aperature
8. Carotid canal internal aperature
9. Foramen lacerum (plugged up with cartilage in life)
10. Mandibular fossa
11. Foramen spinosum
12. Foramen ovale
13. Auditory tube sulcus
14. Vomer
15. Medial and lateral pterygoid plates
16. Pterygoid hamulus
17. Horizontal plate of palatine bone
18. Palatine process of maxillary bone
19. Incisive foramen
20. Major palatine foramen
21. Inferior orbital fissure
22. Inferior nuchal line
23. Superior nuchal line
24. External occipital protuberance (inion)
25. External auditory meatus
26. Petrotympanic fissure

H&N-80 Skull
Inferior aspect
(opposite page)

1 _____
2 _____
3 _____
4 _____
5 _____
6 _____
7 _____
8 _____
9 _____
10 _____
11 _____
12 _____
13 _____
14 _____
15 _____
16 _____
17 _____
18 _____
19 _____
20 _____
21 _____
22 _____
23 _____
24 _____
25 _____
26 _____

T _____
S _____
O _____
Z _____
M _____
P _____
V _____

H&N-81 Autonomic outflow in the head I

(opposite page)

Color and label

1. Ciliary ganglion*
2. Pterygopalatine ganglion*
3. Otic ganglion*
4. Submandibular ganglion*
5. Trigeminal nerve sensory
6. Trigeminal nerve motor root
7. Trigeminal ganglion
8. Nasociliary branch of ophthalmic nerve
9. Long ciliary nerve (sensory to eye)
10. Short ciliary nerve (autonomics)
11. Oculomotor nerve (N III)
12. Oculomotor root to ciliary ganglion (parasympathetics)
13. Sympathetic root to ciliary ganglion
14. Internal carotid artery and plexus
15. Maxillary nerve
16. Pterygopalatine nerves
17. Palatine nerves
18. Posterior lateral nasal nerves
19. Nerve of the pterygoid canal (Vidian nerve)
20. Facial nerve
21. Greater petrosal nerve (branch of facial nerve, N VII)
22. Deep petrosal nerve (sympathetics)
23. Lesser petrosal nerve (branch of glossopharyngeal nerve, N IX)
24. Lingual nerve (branch of mandibular nerve)
25. Chorda tympani nerve (branch of facial nerve)
26. Inferior alveolar nerve (branch of mandibular nerve)
27. Glossopharyngeal nerve (N IX)
28. Vagus nerve (N X)
29. Superior laryngeal branch of vagus nerve
30. Superior cardiac branch of vagus nerve
31. Superior cervical sympathetic ganglion
32. Carotid nerve
33. Middle meningeal artery and plexus
34. Maxillary artery and plexus
35. External carotid artery and plexus
36. Carotid sinus nerve (branch of glossopharyngeal nerve)
37. Carotid sinus
38. Common carotid artery
39. Pharyngeal plexus (nerves X and IX)
40. Superior cervical sympathetic cardiac nerve
41. Auriculotemporal nerve

*These four parasympathetic ganglia contain postganglionic parasympathetic nerve cell bodies upon which preganglionic parasympathetic fibers synapse.

1. _____
2. _____
3. _____
4. _____
5. _____
6. _____
7. _____
8. _____
9. _____
10. _____
11. _____
12. _____
13. _____
14. _____
15. _____
16. _____
17. _____
18. _____
19. _____
20. _____
21. _____
22. _____
23. _____
24. _____
25. _____
26. _____
27. _____
28. _____
29. _____
30. _____
31. _____
32. _____
33. _____
34. _____
35. _____
36. _____
37. _____
38. _____
39. _____
40. _____
41. _____

H&N-81 Autonomic outflow in the head, I

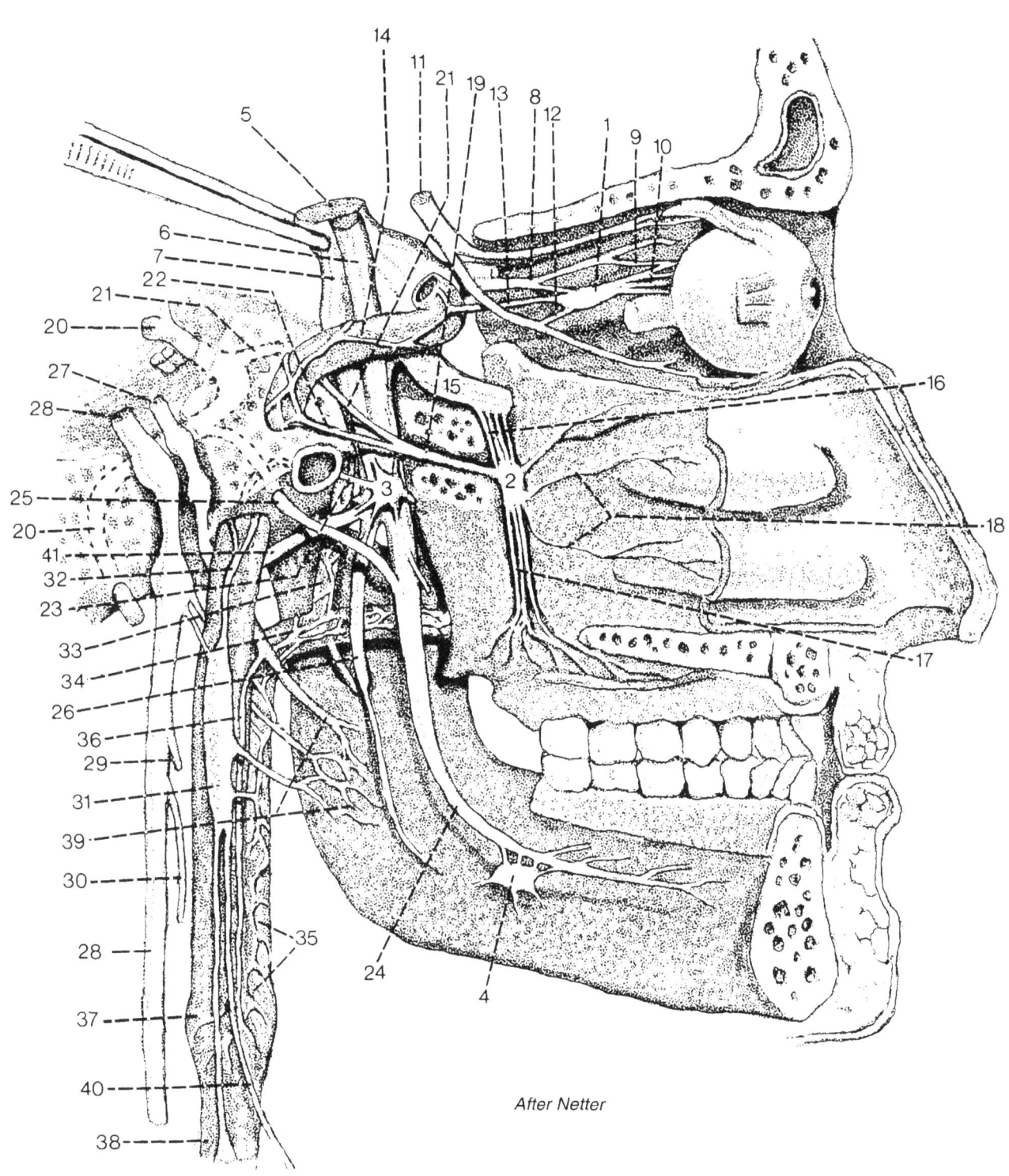

After Netter

H&N-82 Autonomic outflow in the head II
(opposite page)

Color the neurons and trace the paths of their axons

1. Accessory oculomotor nucleus (old name: Edinger-Westfall nucleus) with preganglionic parasympathetic neurons* and fibers (axons)
2. Superior (rostral) salivatory nucleus with preganglionic parasympathetic neurons* and fibers (axons)
3. Inferior (caudal) salivatory nucleus with preganglionic parasympathetic neurons* and fibers (axons)
4. Dorsal nucleus of vagus nerve (dorsal vagal nucleus) with preganglionic parasympathetic neurons* and fibers (axons)
5. Ciliary ganglion with postganglionic parasympathetic neurons giving rise to postganglionic fibers to the constrictor muscles of the iris (these diminish the size of the pupil) and to the circular muscles of the ciliary body (these allow the lens to become more spherical and focus on near objects)
6. Pterygopalatine ganglion with postganglionic parasympathetic neurons giving rise to postganglionic fibers to the lacrimal gland and glands of the nose and palate
7. Otic ganglion with postganglionic parasympathetic neurons giving rise to postganglionic fibers to the parotid gland
8. Submandibular ganglion with postganglionic parasympathetic neurons giving rise to postganglionic fibers to the submandibular and sublingual gland
9. Preganglionic sympathetic nerve cell body in interomediolateral column of thoracic spinal cord
10. Postganglionic sympathetic nerve cell body in superior cervical ganglion
11. Oculomotor nerve (N III)

*Each of the greatly enlarged neurons (or nerve cells) shown here represent hundreds or thousands of microscopic neurons.

12. Inferior branch of oculomotor nerve and oculomotor root to ciliary ganglion
13. Short ciliary nerves
14. Trigeminal nerve (N V)
15. Lacrimal nerve (branch of ophthalmic nerve)
16. Zygomaticofacial branch of maxillary nerve
17. Facial nerve (N VII)
18. Greater petrosal nerve
19. Chorda tympani nerve
20. Glossopharyngeal nerve (N IV)
21. Tympanic nerve and tympanic plexus
22. Lesser petrosal nerve (derived from tympanic plexus)
23. Auriculotemporal nerve (branch of mandibular nerve)
24. Vagus nerve
25. Superior cardiac branch of vagus nerve
26. Postganglionic parasympathetic fiber(s) to eye
27. Postganglionic parasympathetic fiber(s) to lacrimal gland
28. Postganglionic parasympathetic fibers to nasal glands
29. Postganglionic parasympathetic fiber(s) to palatine glands
30. Postganglionic parasympathetic fibers to submandibular and sublingual glands
31. Postganglionic parasympathetic fiber(s) to parotid gland via auriculotemporal nerve
32. Preganglionic parasympathetic fiber(s) to heart
33. Postganglionic sympathetic fiber(s) to nose via carotid plexus and deep petrosal nerve; (sympathetic fibers pass through the parasympathetic ganglion with no interruption)
34. Midbrain
35. Pons
36. Medulla
37. Lacrimal gland
38. Nasal glands and nasal conchae
39. Parotid gland (a small portion)
40. Sublingual gland
41. Submandibular gland

(use abbrevs.)

1. _____
2. _____
3. _____
4. _____
5. _____
6. _____
7. _____
8. _____
9. _____
10. _____
11. _____
12. _____
13. _____
14. _____
15. _____
16. _____
17. _____
18. _____
19. _____
20. _____
21. _____
22. _____
23. _____
24. _____

H&N-82 Autonomic outflow in the head II

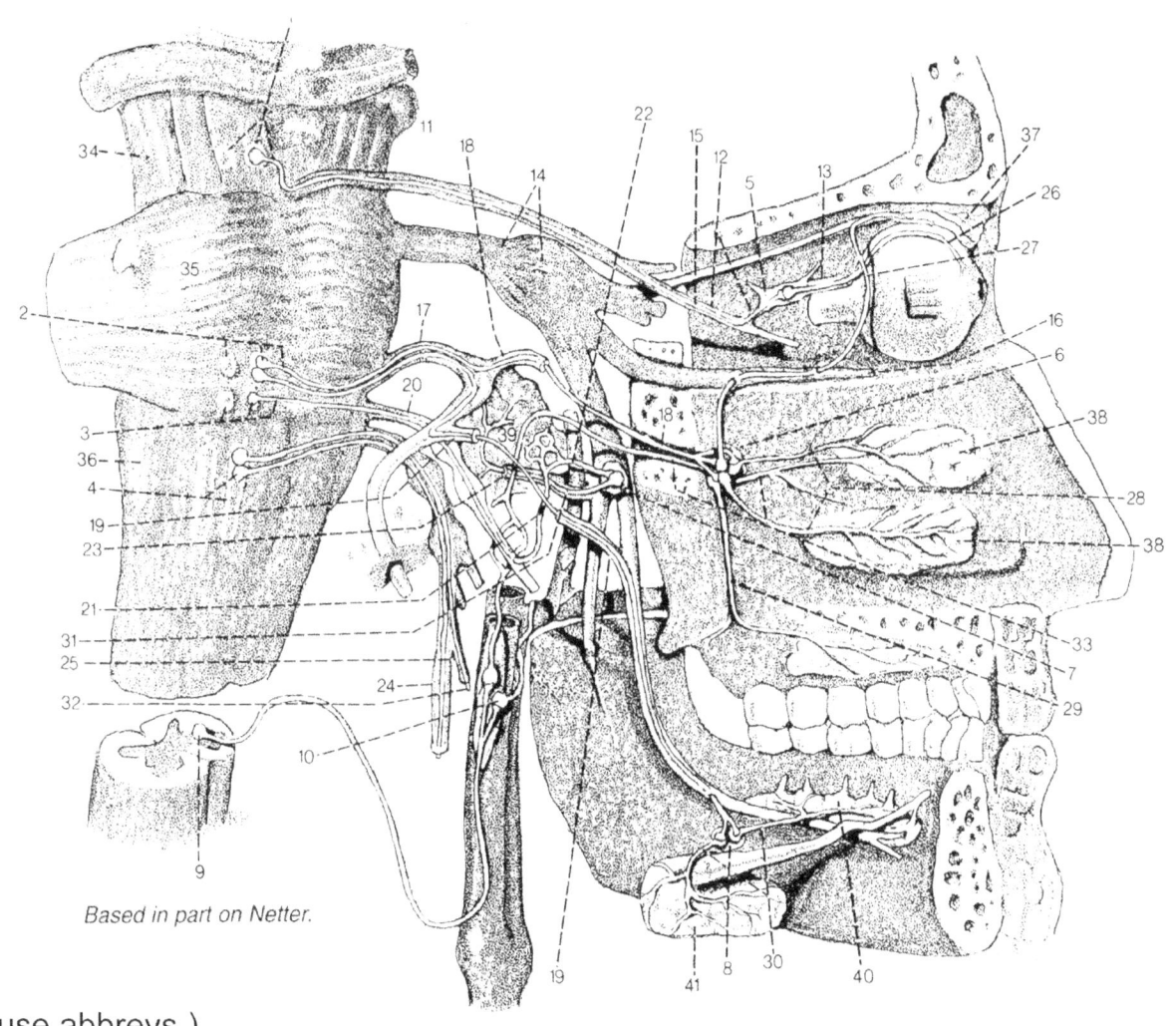

Based in part on Netter.

(use abbrevs.)

25 _____
26 _____
27 _____
28 _____
29 _____
30 _____
31 _____
32 _____
33 _____
34 _____
35 _____
36 _____

37 _____
38 _____
39 _____
40 _____
41 _____

H&N-83 Inferior view of the brain

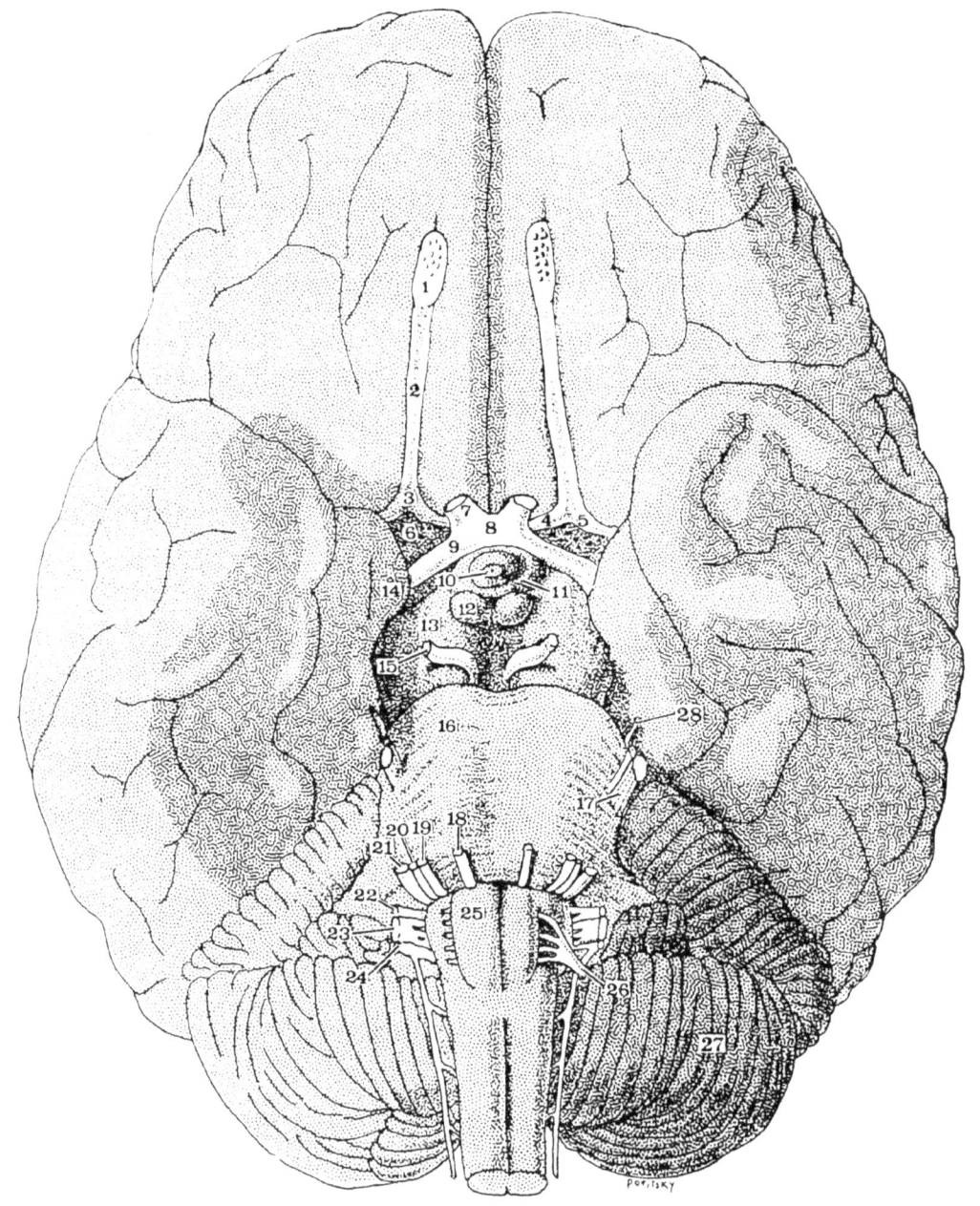

Color* and label

1. Olfactory bulb*
2. Olfactory tract*
3. Olfactory trigone*
4. Medial olfactory stria*
5. Lateral olfactory stria*
6. Anterior perforated substance
7. Optic nerve (cranial nerve II)
8. Optic chiasma*
9. Optic tract*
10. Infundibulum
11. Tuber cinereum
12. Mamillary body
13. Cerebral peduncle
14. Uncus
15. Oculomotor nerve (cranial nerve III)*
16. Pons
17. Trigeminal nerve (cranial nerve V)*
18. Abducent nerve (cranial nerve VI)*
19. Facial nerve (cranial nerve VII) (motor part)*
20. Nervus intermedius (part of facial nerve)*
21. Vestibulocochlear nerve (cranial nerve VIII)*
22. Glossopharyngeal nerve (cranial nerve IX)*
23. Vagus nerve (cranial nerve X)*
24. Accessory nerve (cranial nerve XI)*
25. Pyramids
26. Hypoglossal nerve (cranial nerve XII)*
27. Cerebellum (hemisphere)
28. Trochlear nerve (cranial nerve IV)*

H&N-83 Inferior view of the brain
(opposite page)

1 _____

2 _____

3 _____

4 _____

5 _____

6 _____

7 _____

8 _____

9 _____

10 _____

11 _____

12 _____

13 _____

14 _____

15 _____

16 _____

17 _____

18 _____

19 _____

20 _____

21 _____

22 _____

23 _____

24 _____

25 _____

26 _____

27 _____

28 _____

H&N-84 Medial view of right half of brain

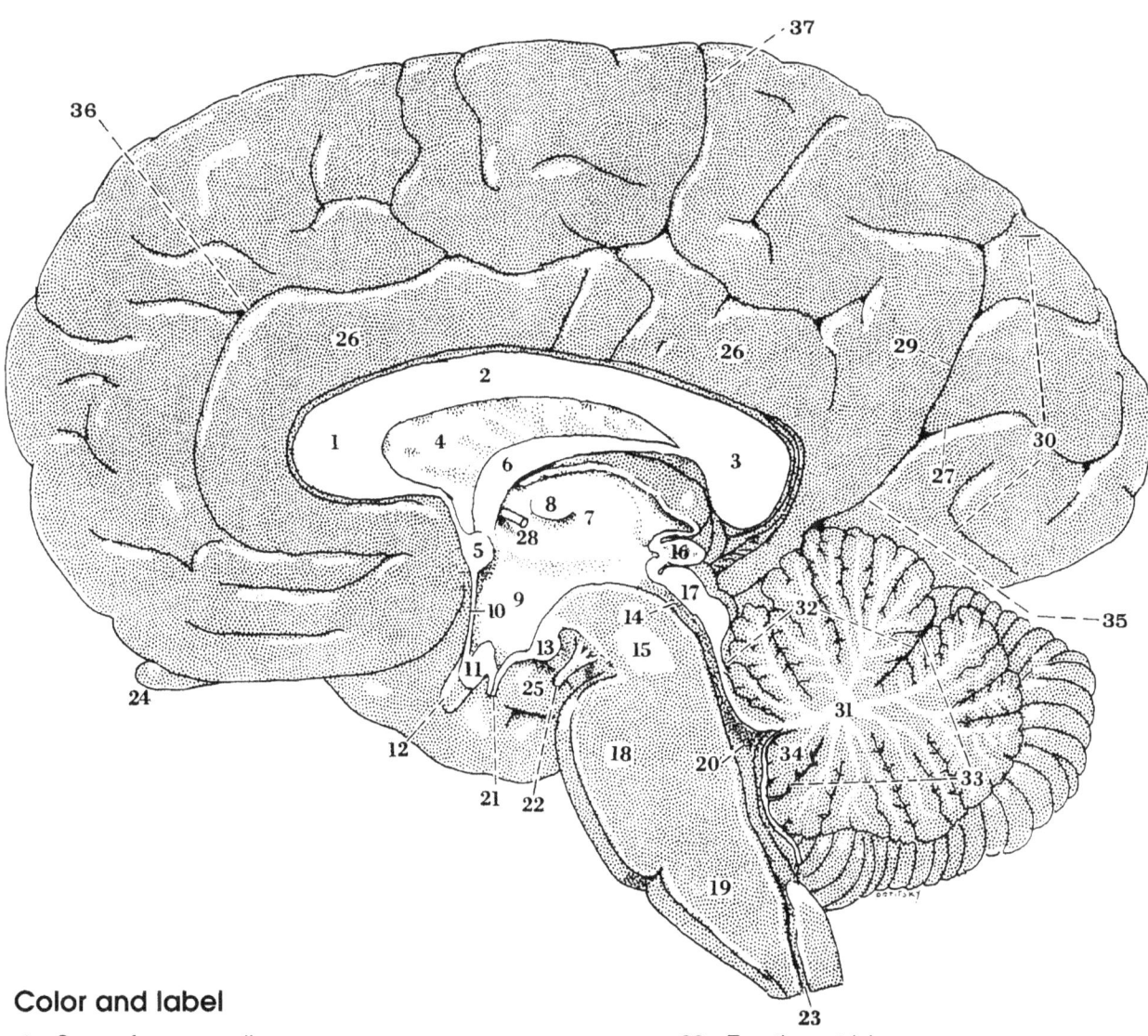

Color and label

1. Genu of corpus callosum
2. Body of corpus callosum
3. Splenium of corpus callosum
4. Septum pellucidum
5. Anterior commissure
6. Fornix
7. Thalamus
8. Interthalamic adhesion
9. Hypothalamus
10. Lamina terminalis
11. Optic chiasm
12. Optic nerve
13. Mamillary body
14. Cerebral aqueduct
15. Decussation of superior cerebellar peduncles
16. Pineal body
17. Mesencephalic tectum (formerly lamina quadrigemina)
18. Pons
19. Medulla
20. Fourth ventricle
21. Infundibulum
22. Oculomotor nerve
23. Central canal of spinal cord
24. Olfactory bulb
25. Uncus of temporal lobe
26. Cingulate gyrus
27. Calcarine sulcus
28. Probe in interventricular foramen
29. Parieto-occipital sulcus
30. Occipital lobe
31. White matter of vermis
32. Anterior lobe of cerebellum
33. Posterior lobe of cerebellum
34. Nodulus of cerebellum
35. Common stem of parieto-occipital sulcus and calcarine sulcus
36. Cingulate sulcus
37. Marginal part of cingulate sulcus

H&N-84 Medial view of right half of brain
(opposite page)

1 _____
2 _____
3 _____
4 _____
5 _____
6 _____
7 _____
8 _____
9 _____
10 _____
11 _____
12 _____
13 _____
14 _____
15 _____
16 _____
17 _____
18 _____
19 _____

20 _____
21 _____
22 _____
23 _____
24 _____
25 _____
26 _____
27 _____
28 _____
29 _____
30 _____
31 _____
32 _____
33 _____
34 _____
35 _____
36 _____
37 _____

H&N-85 The cranial nerves

Ventral aspect of brain stem showing exit of cranial nerves.
There are twelve pairs of cranial nerves. They are numbered with Roman numerals (just like the successive Super Bowls!).

Color and label (unlabelled side)

Cranial nerve I is the **olfactory nerve** (Latin, *olfacia*, to smell). It is made up of the axons of bipolar olfactory receptors in the roof of the nasal cavity. These axons group into about 20 bundles called fila that penetrate the cribriform plate of the ethmoid bone and end in the olfactory bulb. The axons of the olfactory nerve are thin and unmyelinated and are easily broken should the olfactory bulb be raised.

Cranial nerve II is the **optic nerve**. It consists of about one million axons that arise from the ganglion cells in the retina. The optic nerve is the only nerve that is enclosed by the three meninges, the dura mater, arachnoid mater, and the pia mater.

Cranial nerve III is the **oculomotor nerve**. It supplies motor fibers and movement to four extrabulbar eye muscles and the raiser of the eyelid (levator palpebrae). By convention the optic nerve is named "optic nerve" from the eyeball to the optic chiasm; from the chiasm to its termination in the lateral geniculate body it is called "optic tract."

Cranial nerve IV is the **trochlear nerve** (Greek, *trochlea*, pulley). It supplies only one extrabulbar muscle, the superior oblique. It is the only cranial nerve that becomes completely crossed (it supplies the opposite superior oblique). It also is the only cranial nerve that exits from the dorsal aspect of the brain stem.

Cranial nerve V is the **trigeminal nerve** (Latin, *trigeminus*, threefold). It is mainly sensory and divides into three large branches, the ophthalmic nerve, the maxillary nerve, and the mandibular nerve. These three nerves supply the face, eye, nose, mouth, teeth, and the anterior two-thirds of the tongue with pain, touch, and temperature sensibilities. It has a smaller motor component that travels with the mandibular nerve and supplies the muscles of the jaw (muscles of mastication).

Cranial nerve VI is the **abducent nerve** (Latin, *abducere*, to lead away). It supplies only one extrabulbar eye muscle, the lateral rectus which turns the eye lateral.

Cranial nerve VII is the **facial nerve**. It arises by two roots. The larger motor root supplies the muscles of facial expression. Immediate lateral to the motor root is the smaller root, the **nervus intermedius**. The nervus intermedius contains taste fibers from the anterior two-thirds of the tongue and parasympathetic fibers that supply the lacrimal gland, nasal glands, submandibular gland, and sublingual gland.

Cranial nerve VIII is the **vestibulocochlear nerve**. It carries two distinct sensory modalities from the inner ear. The older vestibular portion carries information about the position and movement of the head. The vestibular part of the inner ear responds to the head being turned, tilted, or accelerated in a straight line. The newer cochlear portion of the vestibulocochlear carries hearing sensibility from the cochlea to the medial geniculate body.

Cranial nerve IX is the **glossopharyngeal nerve** (Greek, literally "tongue-throat"). It is mainly sensory to the upper pharynx and soft palate. It supplies pain, touch, temperature, and taste to the posterior one-third of the tongue. It supplies motor fibers that join with those of the vagus nerve to form the pharyngeal plexus, which innervates the soft palate and upper pharynx. Parasympathetic fibers in the glossopharyngeal nerve supply the parotid gland.

Cranial nerve X is the **vagus nerve**. It contains five different kinds of fibers. These include preganglionic parasympathetic fibers that innervate the esophagus, heart, lungs, stomach, and intestines. Numerous visceral afferent (incoming) fibers function in cardiac and pulmonary reflexes. The vagus supplies motor control of the pharynx and larynx. Taste fibers from taste buds on the epiglottis travel within the vagus nerve, as do a few afferent fibers from the skin of the ear.

Cranial nerve XI is the **accessory nerve** (old name, spinal accessory nerve). It arises by two roots, a cranial one from the medulla and a spinal one from the cervical spinal cord. It supplies only two muscles, the trapezius and the sternocleidomastoid.

Cranial nerve XII is the **hypoglossal nerve**. It supplies all the homolateral tongue muscles (on the same side).

H&N-85 The cranial nerves

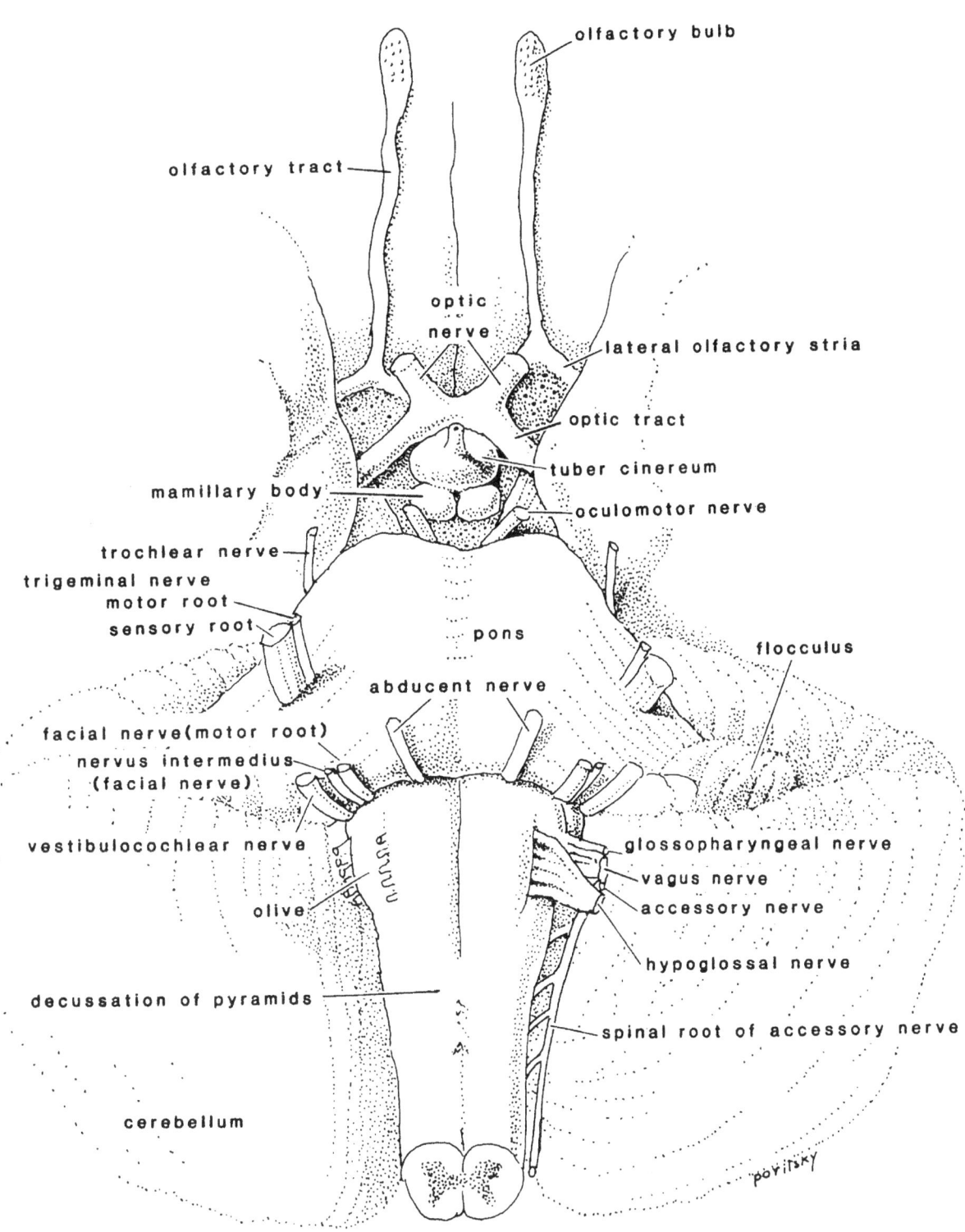

H&N-86 Brain stem

Dorsal aspect
(opposite page)

Color and label

1. Cavity of septum pellucidum
2. Corpus callosum (a small section)
3. Septum pellucidum
4. Internal capsule
5. Putamen
6. Stria terminalis and thalamostriate vein
7. Tail of caudate nucleus
8. Ventricle III
9. Choroid membrane (tela choroidea) of third ventricle
10. Pineal gland
11. Brachium of inferior colliculus
12. Inferior colliculus
13. Trochlear nerve (originated from opposite trochlear nucleus)
14. Superior cerebellar peduncle
15. Facial colliculus
16. Vestibular area
17. Lateral aperature of fourth ventricle (IV)
18. Hypoglossal trigone
19. Vagal trigone
20. Obex (caudal angle of ventricle IV)
21. Fasciculus gracilis
22. Fasciculus cuneatus
23. Posterior intermediate sulcus
24. Posterior median sulcus
25. Tubercle of nucleus cuneatus
26. Tubercle of nucleus gracilis
27. Tenia of ventricle IV (line of attachment of choroid membrane to rim of ventricle IV)
28. Accessory nerve (N XI)
29. Vagus nerve (N X)
30. Glossopharyngeal nerve (N IX)
31. Stria medularis of ventricle IV
32. Inferior cerebellar peduncle (old name, restiform body)
33. Middle cerebellum peduncle (old name, brachium pontis)
34. Superior medullary velum
35. Trigeminal nerve (N V)
36. Superior colliculus
37. Medial geniculate body
38. Lateral geniculate body
39. Habenular triangle
40. Internal capsule (sublenticular part)
41. Thalamus
42. Fornix (body; cut)
43. Caudate nucleus (body)
44. Lateral ventricle (left)
45. Caudate nucleus (head)

1 _____
2 _____
3 _____
4 _____
5 _____
6 _____
7 _____
8 _____
9 _____
10 _____
11 _____
12 _____
13 _____
14 _____
15 _____
16 _____

17 _____
18 _____
19 _____
20 _____
21 _____
22 _____
23 _____
24 _____
25 _____
26 _____
27 _____
28 _____
29 _____
30 _____
31 _____
32 _____

33 _____
34 _____
35 _____
36 _____
37 _____
38 _____
39 _____
40 _____
41 _____
42 _____
43 _____
44 _____
45 _____

H&N-86 Brain stem

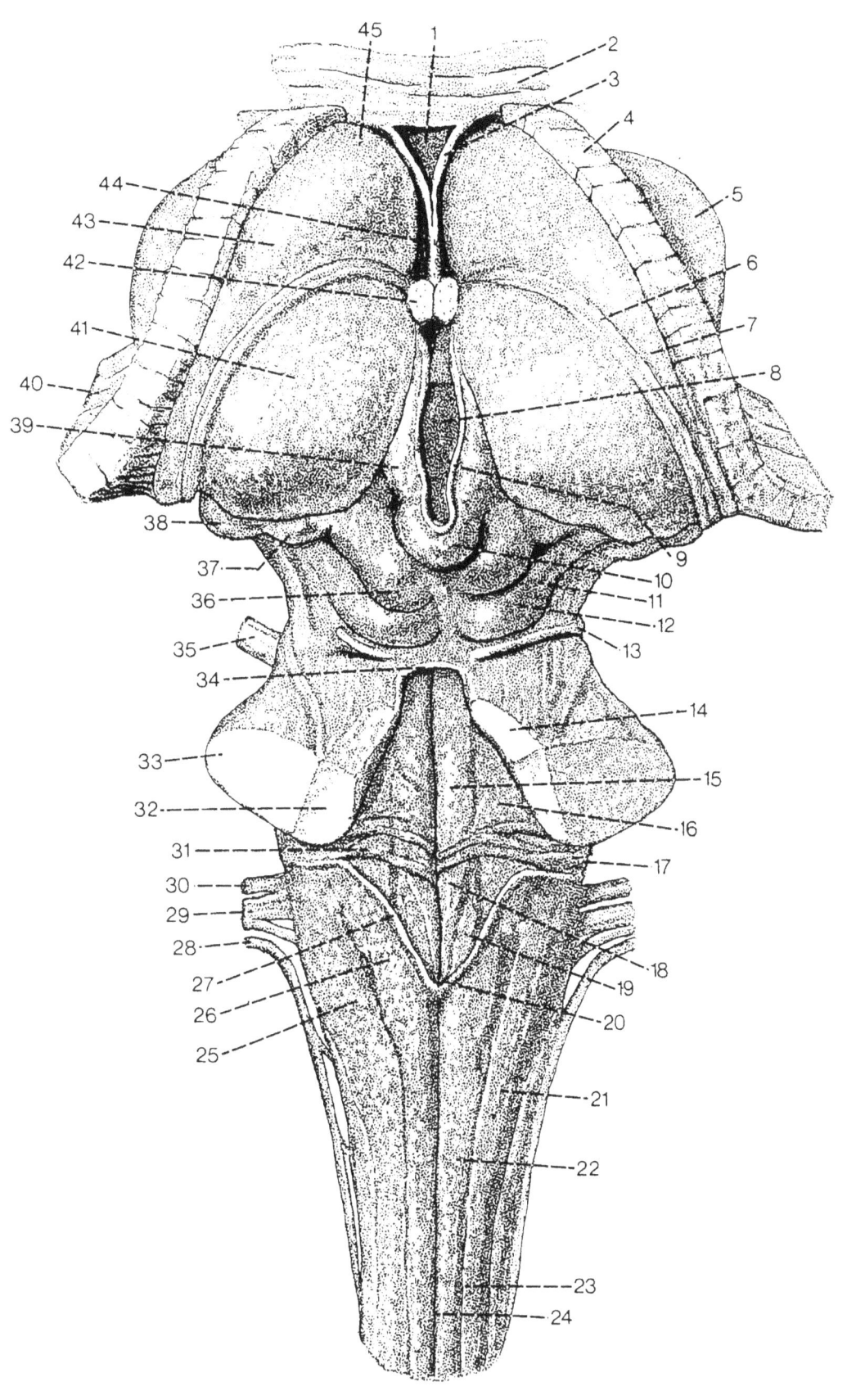

H&N-87 Arterial supply at base of brain

Anterior aspect
(opposite page)

Color and label

1. Vertebral arteries (right and left)*
2. Internal carotid arteries (right and left)*
3. Anterior spinal artery
4. Basilar artery (formed by the union of the two vertebral arteries)
5. Posterior inferior cerebellar artery
6. Anterior inferior cerebellar artery
7. Labyrinthine artery
8. Superior cerebellar artery
9. Posterior cerebral artery
10. Posterior communicating artery
11. Middle cerebral artery
12. Anterior cerebral artery (note its course in the longitudinal cerebral fissure as it curves around the genu of the corpus callosum)
13. Anterior communicating artery (prone to aneurysms)
14. Branch of the posterior cerebral artery
15. Pontine branches off basilar artery

*These four arteries, the right and left vertebral arteries and the right and left internal carotid arteries, are the sole supply of arterial blood to the brain.

1 _____
2 _____
3 _____
4 _____
5 _____
6 _____
7 _____
8 _____
9 _____
10 _____
11 _____
12 _____
13 _____
14 _____
15 _____

H&N-87 Arterial supply at base of brain

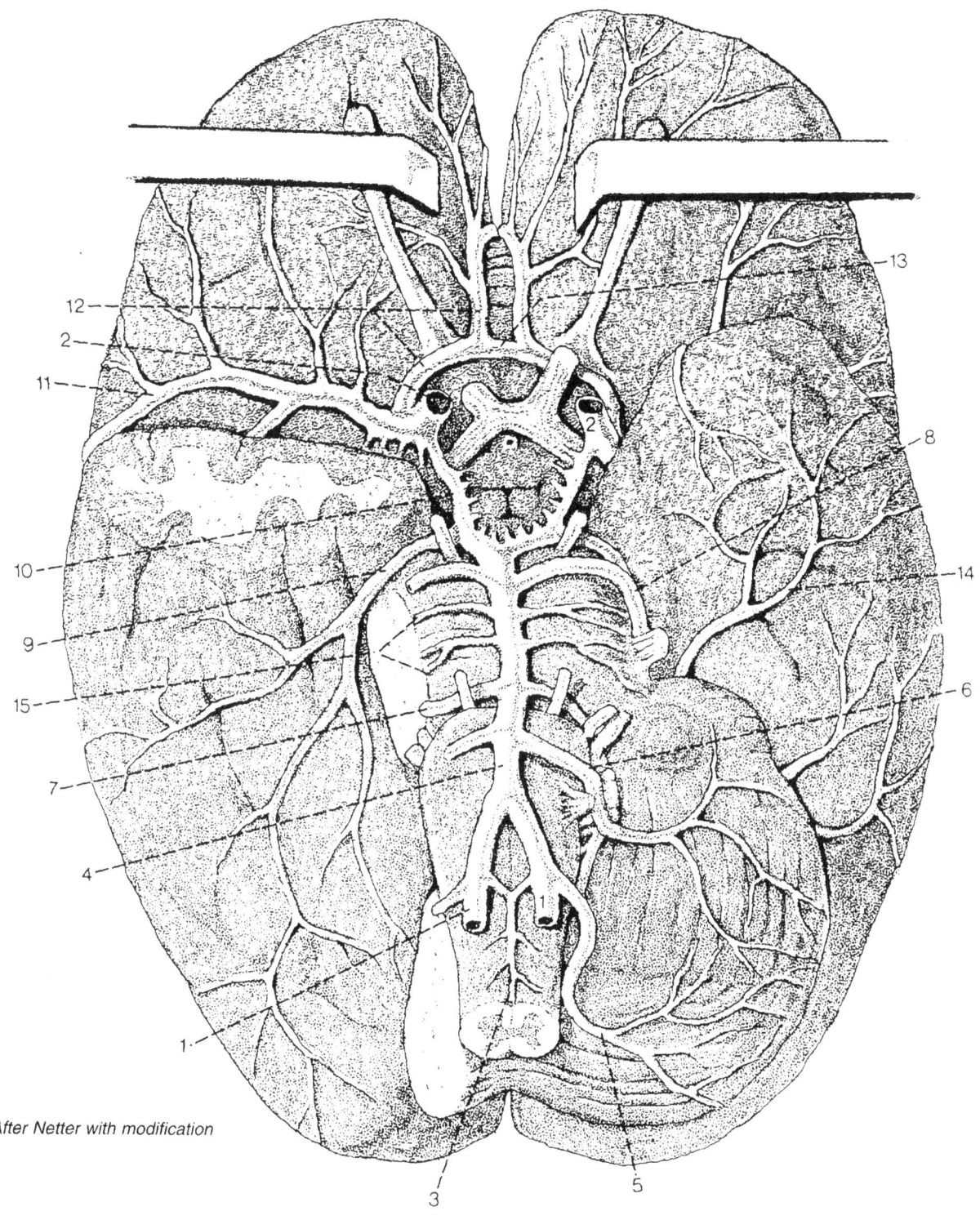

After Netter with modification

147

Thalamus means bedroom
Etymological cartoon

Thalamus meant bedroom or inner chamber in both Latin and Greek. Why the thalamus, which is a solid mass of neurons, should be named a room or chamber is something of a mystery. It probably goes back to the ancients' belief that hollow chambers in the brain stored particles of sensation conveyed to the brain by hollow nerves. The optic nerve supposedly carried particles of vision to its chamber, the optic thalamus. A careful examination of the brain would have revealed to the ancients that the lateral geniculate body, which is that part of the thalamus where the optic nerve ends, is not hollow but rather solid; nor is any other part of the thalamus hollow. Unfortunately the ancients' knowledge of brain anatomy was founded more on doctrine than on actual dissection and examination. For a long time the term **optic thalamus** was used for the thalamus, even after it was shown that it was solid, not hollow. Eventually "optic" was discarded and the name was shortened to simply thalamus.

Pituitary gland. At one time the pituitary gland was believed to secrete phlegm. Its name is derived from the Latin *pituita*, which means phlegm. Pituita itself is an onomatope, which means it is imitative of the sound associated with it, which in this case is the sound of spitting, much like our expression "ptooey." The ancients thought that the brain extracted phlegm from the blood. The phlegm was then funneled into the pituitary gland. In fact, the name of the pituitary stalk, **infundibulum**, means funnel in Latin. From the pituitary gland the phlegm was supposedly conveyed to the roof of the nose, where it migrated through tiny holes in the cribriform plate into the nose.

Ostium (Latin) meant door. It is now used in anatomy for a small opening of a vessel. It is derived from *os* (mouth).

Tectum (Latin) was either a ceiling or a roof. The tectum is that part of the midbrain dorsal to the cerebral aqueduct. The former name for the tectum was **lamina quadrigemina**, the "plate with the quadruplets," that is, the four colliculi.

Colliculus (Latin) meant little hill, from *collis*, hill.
Folia (Latin) meant leaves. One leaf was a **folium**. The transverse folds of the cerebellar cortex are called folia.
Ramus (Latin) meant branch.
Arbor (Latin) meant tree. The **arbor vitae**, "tree of life," was the old name for the white matter in the cerebellum.
Dendrite is derived from the Greek **dendron** (tree) and means little tree or tree-like.
Radix (Latin) meant root. **Radicular** relates to a root. **Radiculitis** means inflammation of a nerve root. A **radical** change is a change so drastic that it gets down to the roots, and may even pull out the roots!
Funiculus (Latin) is derived from **funis** (rope) and meant little rope or string. The white matter of the spinal cord is divided into three funiculi.
Pulivinus (Latin) meant a cushion. **Pulivinar** meant couch. The pulivinar of the thalamus resembles a cushion.
Kline was a bed in ancient Greece. Words such as **clinic, recline, incline** all come from this root. A **clinician** was originally one who visited and treated patients at the bedside.
Murus (Latin) was a wall. **Intramural** ganglia are groups of nerve cells within the walls of the heart, the intestines, and other viscera. **Intramural** sports are held within the walls of the school or college.
Clinoid process means bed post, being derived from kline (bed). The four clinoid processes are found in the skull, where they make up part of the **sella turcica**, or "Turkish saddle," which holds the pituitary gland.

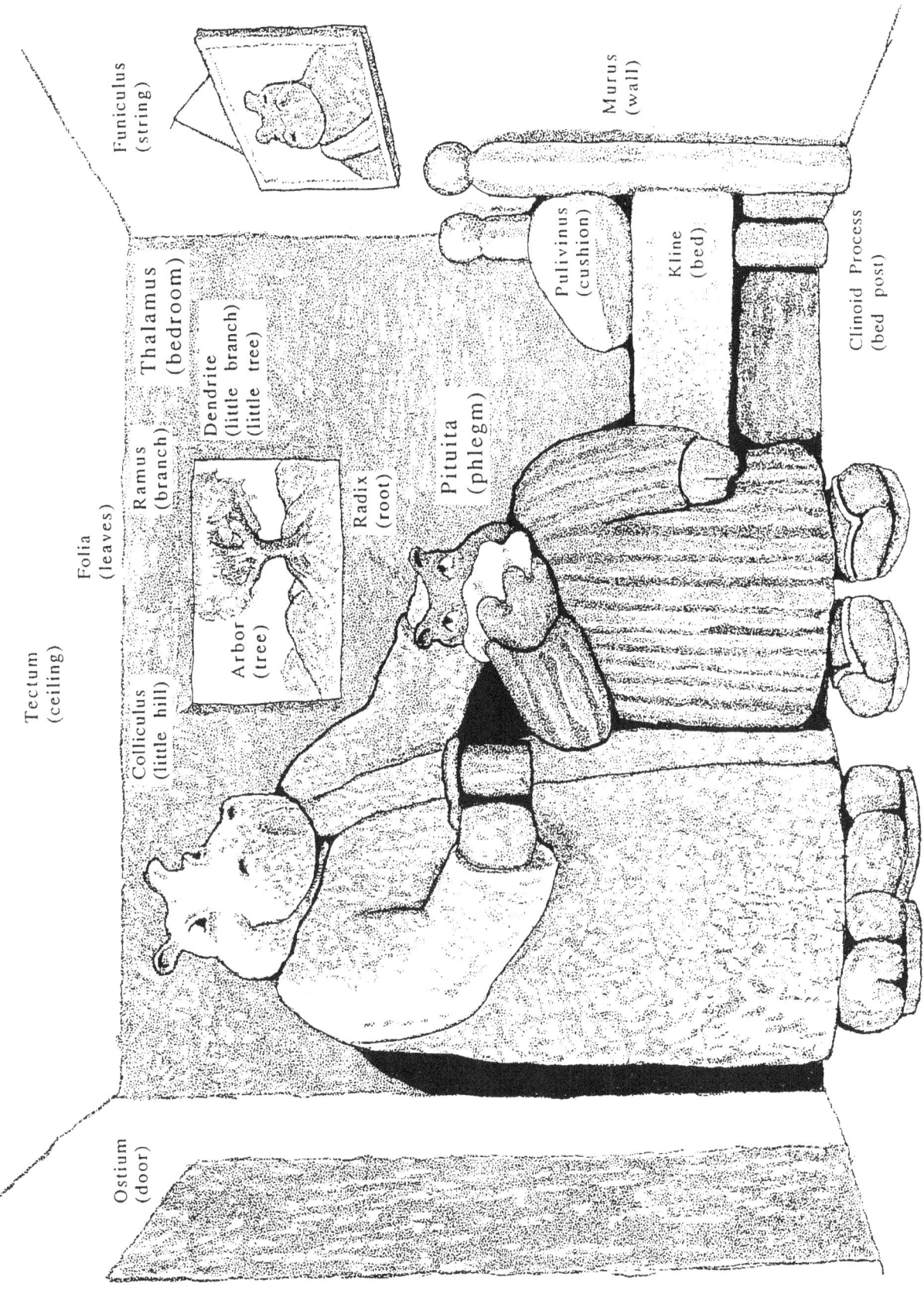

H&N-88 Head frontal section; level of eyes and nasal cavity

Viewed from the front

Color and label

1. Skin of scalp
2. Frontal diploic vein
3. Frontal bone
4. Bone of frontal crest
5. Frontal lobe of brain
6. Galea aponeurotica (epicranial aponeurosis); extends from frontalis muscle anteriorly to occipitalis muscle posteriorly
7. Loose connective tissue layer of scalp
8. Frontal branch of superficial temporal vein
9. Terminal branch of frontopolar artery (branch of anterior cerebral artery)
10. Frontal sinuses (right and left)
11. Supraorbital nerve
12. Superior ophthalmic vein
13. Superior rectus muscle (tendon)
14. Tendon of superior oblique muscle within trochlea
15. Lacrimal gland
16. Sclera of eye
17. Choroid layer of eye (dark pigmented layer)
18. Crista galli
19. Nasal cavities and left middle nasal concha
20. Maxillary sinus
21. Nasal septum (perpendicular plate of ethmoid above, septal cartilage and vomer below)
22. Levator labii superioris muscle (facial expression)
23. Superior alveolar nerve (left)
24. Anterior nasal spine
25. Maxilla
26. Root and pulp cavity of upper left canine in maxilla
27. Facial artery (above), superior labial artery (below)
28. Buccinator muscle
29. Submandibular ducts opening in sublingual papillae (caruncles)
30. Inferior labial artery
31. Hyoglossus muscle
32. Mentalis muscle
33. Superior alveolar nerves and artery (right)
34. Infraorbital nerve
35. Inferior nasal concha and inferior nasal meatus (beneath and lateral to inferior nasal concha)
36. Middle nasal concha
37. Inferior oblique muscle
38. Ethmoid air cells (sinuses)
39. Nasolacrimal duct
40. Superficial temporal vein and artery (frontal branch)
41. Anterior temporal diploic veins
42. Tendon of levator palpebrae superioris muscle
43. Orbital fat
44. Terminal branch of sphenopalatine artery in incisive canal

1 _____
2 _____
3 _____
4 _____
5 _____
6 _____
7 _____
8 _____
9 _____
10 _____
11 _____
12 _____
13 _____
14 _____

15 _____
16 _____
17 _____
18 _____
19 _____
20 _____
21 _____
22 _____
23 _____
24 _____
25 _____
26 _____
27 _____
28 _____

H&N-88 Head frontal section; level of eyes and nasal cavity

Viewed from the front

29 _____
30 _____
31 _____
32 _____
33 _____
34 _____
35 _____
36 _____
37 _____
38 _____
39 _____
40 _____
41 _____
42 _____
43 _____
44 _____

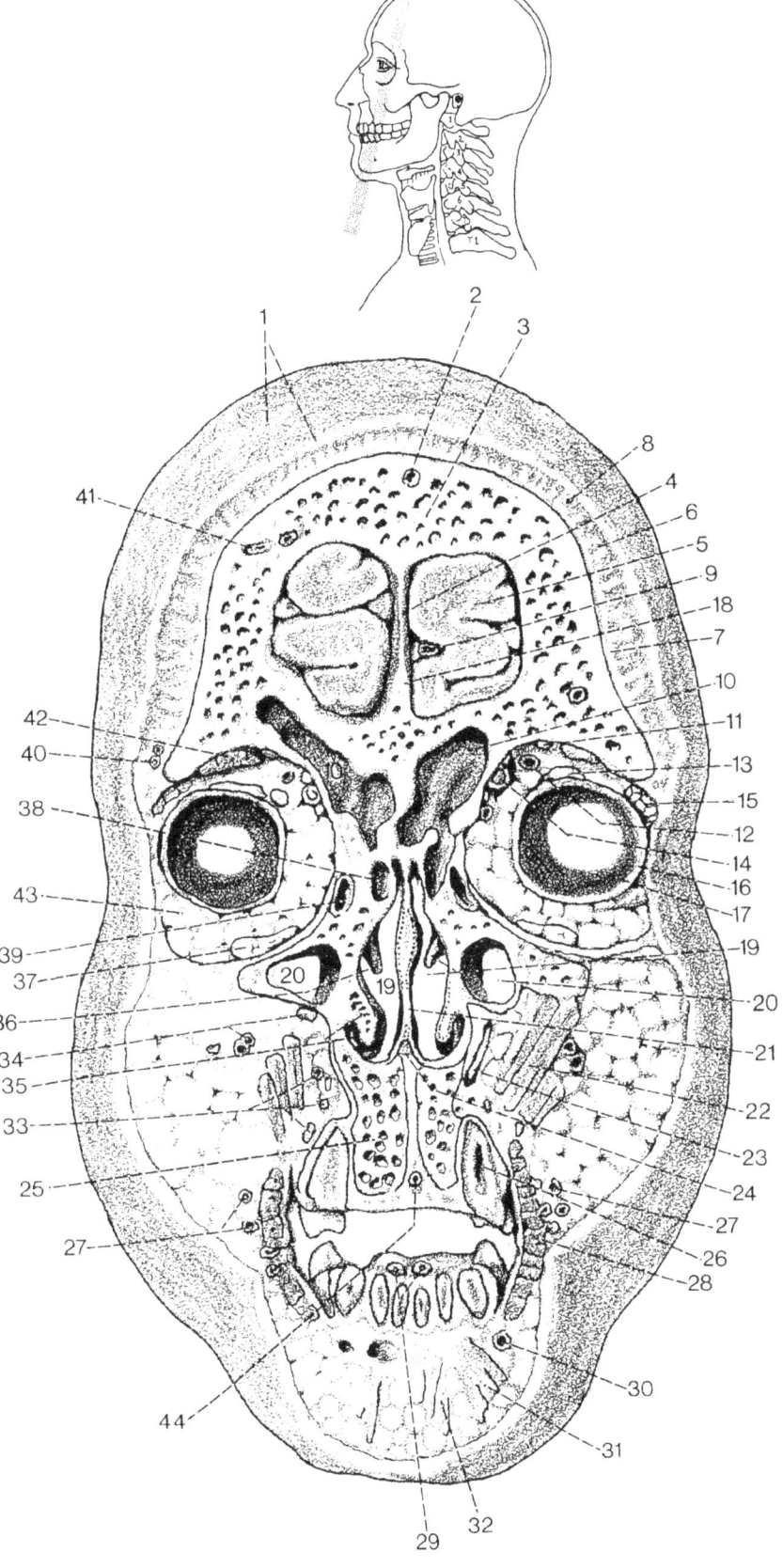

151

H&N-89 Eye muscles, sinuses level

Color and label

1. Falx cerebri
2. Superior sagittal sinus
3. Dura mater
4. Diploic veins
5. Superior frontal gyrus
6. Middle frontal gyrus
7. Anterior temporal diploic vein
8. Inferior frontal gyrus
9. Gyrus rectus (straight gyrus)
10. Superficial temporal artery (frontal branch)
11. Supraorbital nerve and artery
12. Superficial temporal vein (frontal branch)
13. Lacrimal nerve
14. Superior rectus and levator palpebrae muscles
15. Superior ophthalmic vein and ophthalmic artery
16. Fundus of eye (back portion)—retina (inner gray) and choroid layer (dark pigmented middle coat)
17. Sclera of eye (outer white fibrous coat of eyeball)
18. Superior oblique muscle (above), medial rectus muscle (below)
19. Inferior rectus muscle and inferior division of oculomotor nerve
20. Infraorbital nerve and infraorbital artery
21. Ethmoid bone (orbital plate—lamina papyracea)
22. Ethmoid air cells (sinuses)
23. Middle nasal concha and middle nasal meatus (space)
24. Maxillary sinus
25. Nasal septum (perpindicular plate of ethmoid bone above and vomer below)
26. Greater palatine artery and nerve
27. Facial nerve—buccal branches
28. Hard palate (maxillary portion) and glands in mucosa of hard palate
29. Buccinator muscle
30. Buccal branch of facial nerve
31. Facial artery
32. Labial arteries and mandibular branches of facial nerve
33. Platysma muscle
34. Submandibular duct and sublingual gland
35. Inferior alveolar nerve in mandible
36. Genioglossus muscle
37. Mandible
38. Submental veins
39. Sublingual vein (in sublingual gland) and inferior alveolar nerve in mandibular canal
40. Tongue
41. Oral cavity
42. Root of tooth in mandible
43. Facial artery and buccal branches of facial nerve
44. Root of tooth in maxilla
45. Facial vein and buccal branches of facial nerve
46. Inferior nasal concha (turbinate) and inferior nasal meatus (space)
47. Nasal cavity
48. Infraorbital vein, nerve, and artery
49. Inferior rectus extraocular muscle
50. Orbital fat
51. Lateral rectus extraocular muscle
52. Zygomatic bone
53. Medial rectus extraocular muscle
54. Optic nerve
55. Lacrimal gland
56. Superior oblique muscle (medial), superior rectus muscle, levator palpebrae muscle (directly above superior rectus)
57. Crista galli (in midline) and cribriform plate (both part of ethmoid bone)
58. Medial orbitofrontal artery (branch of anterior cerebral artery)
59. Frontopolar artery (branch of anterior cerebral artery)
60. Frontal bone
61. Branches of ascending frontal artery (candelabra artery) of middle cerebral artery
62. Cerebral cortex (gray matter)—contains 6 layers of nerve cell bodies
63. White matter (largely myelinated axons)

1 _____
2 _____
3 _____
4 _____
5 _____
6 _____
7 _____
8 _____
9 _____
10 _____
11 _____
12 _____
13 _____
14 _____
15 _____
16 _____
17 _____
18 _____
19 _____
20 _____
21 _____
22 _____
23 _____
24 _____
25 _____
26 _____
27 _____
28 _____
29 _____
30 _____
31 _____
32 _____
33 _____
34 _____
35 _____
36 _____
37 _____
38 _____
39 _____

40 _____
41 _____
42 _____
43 _____
44 _____
45 _____
46 _____
47 _____
48 _____
49 _____
50 _____
51 _____
52 _____
53 _____
54 _____
55 _____
56 _____
57 _____
58 _____
59 _____
60 _____
61 _____
62 _____
63 _____

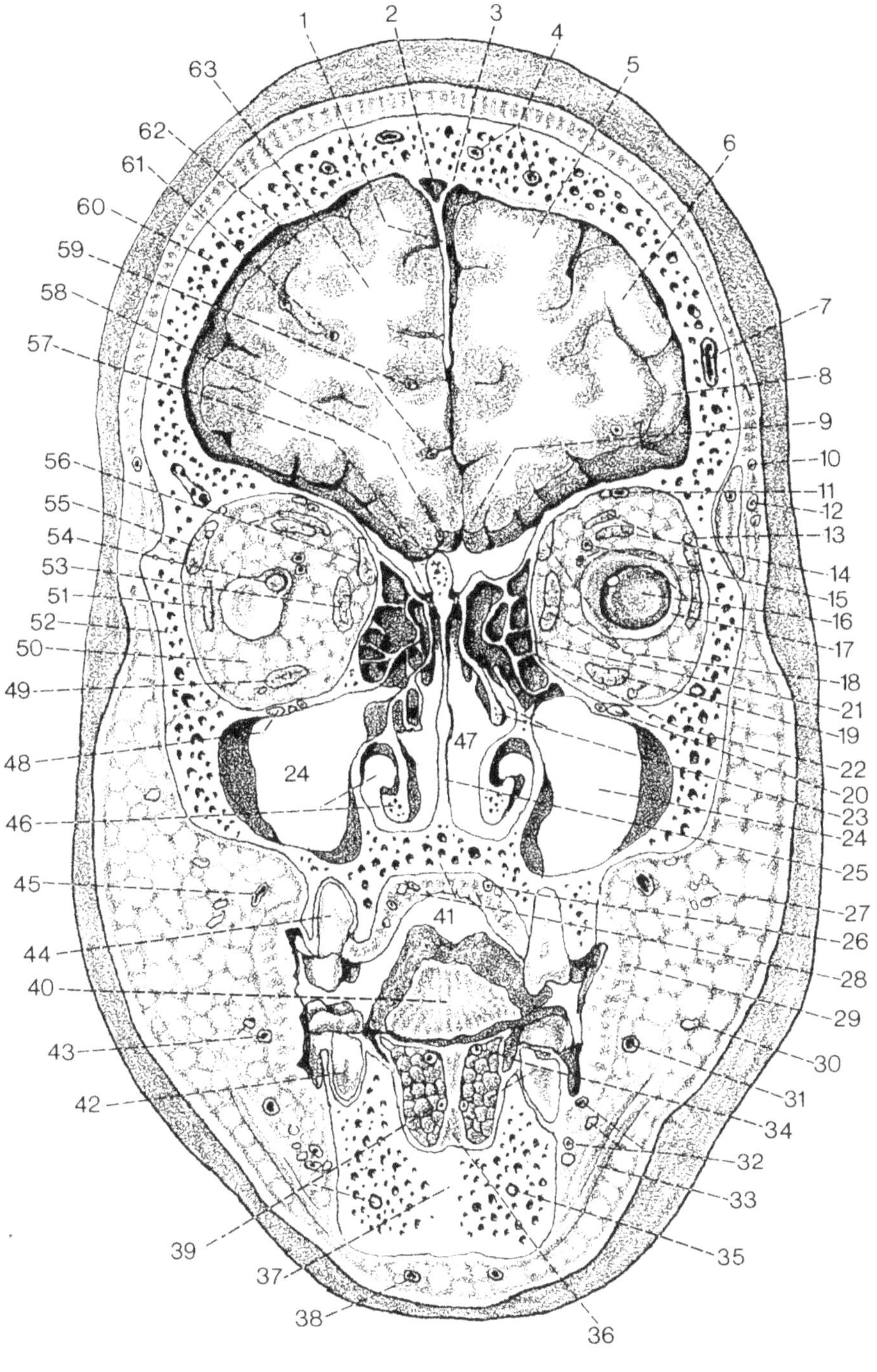

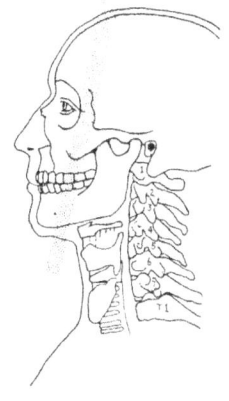

H&N-90 Maxillary sinuses level

Color and label

1. Superior sagittal sinus
2. Longitudinal cerebral fissure (space between cerebral hemispherres)
3. Callosomarginal artery (branch of anterior cerebral artery)
4. Superior frontal gyrus
5. Anterior cerebral arteries curving upwards in front genu of corpus callosum (become pericallosal arteries)
6. Frontal bone
7. Frontal tributary of superficial temporal vein
8. Middle frontal gyrus
9. Anterior temporal diploic vein
10. Straight gyrus (gyrus rectus) of frontal lobe
11. Orbital gyrus of frontal lobe
12. Inferior frontal gyrus
13. Lateral orbitofrontal artery (branch of middle cerebral artery)
14. Levator palpebrae superioris muscle, frontal nerve, superior rectus muscle
15. Superior ophthalmic vein (medial), lacrimal nerve (lateral)
16. Superficial temporal vein and artery
17. Optic nerve in optic canal, ophthalmic artery (immediately above the nerve), lateral rectus muscle
18. Superior oblique muscle (above), medial rectus muscle (immediately below)
19. Inferior rectus muscle, infraorbital nerve (in infraorbital groove in floor of orbit)
20. Temporalis muscle
21. Zygomatic arch
22. Ethmoid air cells (sinuses)
23. Left maxillary sinus
24. Masseter muscle (a small portion)
25. Inferior nasal concha (turbinate), inferior nasal meatus
26. Parotid duct, buccal branches of facial nerve
27. Greater palatine artery and nerve (branch of maxillary nerve in mucosa of hard palate)
28. Molar teeth in maxilla (above) and mandible (below)
29. Buccinator muscle, facial vein
30. Septum of tongue, dorsal lingual vein
31. Facial artery, mandibular branches of facial nerve
32. Inferior alveolar nerve, vein, and artery in mandibular canal
33. Submandibular duct immediately above lingual nerve
34. Genioglossus muscle, deep lingual vein
35. Hypoglossal nerve (above), sublingual branch of lingual artery (below)
36. Mylohyoid muscle, mylohyoid nerve
37. Anterior belly of digastric muscle (left)
38. Sublingual gland
39. Submental vein
40. Geniohyoid muscles (right and left)
41. Genioglossus muscle (right side)
42. Anterior belly of right digastric muscle
43. Hypoglossal nerve medial to lingual artery
44. Sublingual gland
45. Inferior alveolar nerve, vein, artery in mandibular canal
46. Facial artery and mandibular branch(es) of facial nerve
47. Submandibular duct (lingual nerve just below)
48. Mandible
49. Buccinator muscle, facial vein
50. Lingual mucosa on dorsum of tongue
51. Oral cavity
52. Parotid duct (buccal branches of facial nerve)
53. Glands of hard palate
54. Right maxillary sinus
55. Right nasal cavity
56. Left nasal cavity
57. Zygomatic arch
58. Middle nasal concha, middle nasal meatus
59. Lateral rectus muscle
60. Lacrimal nerve (lateral), frontal nerve (medial)
61. Greater wing of sphenoid bone
62. Orbital plate of frontal bone
63. Medial orbitofrontal artery and olfactory tract
64. Anterior cerebral arteries
65. Anterior temporal diploic vein
66. Frontal lobe of cerebral hemisphere (white matter)
67. Cingulate gyrus
68. Galea aponeurotica (epicranial aponeurosis)
69. Cingulate sulcus
70. Falx cerebri
71. Lingual artery
72. Buccal fat pad

1 _____
2 _____
3 _____
4 _____
5 _____
6 _____
7 _____
8 _____
9 _____
10 _____
11 _____
12 _____
13 _____
14 _____
15 _____
16 _____
17 _____
18 _____
19 _____
20 _____
21 _____
22 _____
23 _____
24 _____
25 _____
26 _____
27 _____
28 _____
29 _____
30 _____
31 _____
32 _____
33 _____

34 _____
35 _____
36 _____
37 _____
38 _____
39 _____
40 _____
41 _____
42 _____
43 _____
44 _____
45 _____
46 _____
47 _____
48 _____
49 _____
50 _____
51 _____
52 _____
53 _____
54 _____
55 _____
56 _____
57 _____
58 _____
59 _____
60 _____
61 _____
62 _____
63 _____
64 _____
65 _____

66 _____
67 _____
68 _____
69 _____
70 _____
71 _____
72 _____

H&N-91 Sphenoid sinuses level

Color and label

1. Superior sagittal sinus
2. Subarachnoid space (contains cerebrospinal fluid, traversed by arachnoid trabeculae)—usually is obliterated after death by arachnoid mater separating from dura mater and collapsing on pia mater
3. Falx cerebri
4. Callosomarginal artery (branch of anterior cerebral)
5. Pericallosal artery (continuation of anterior cerebral artery)
6. Anterior temporal diploic vein
7. Corpus callosum (genu)
8. Lateral ventricle (left)
9. Caudate nucleus (head) abutting lateral ventricle
10. Parietal branch of middle cerebral artery
11. Lateral (Sylvian) fissure
12. Superficial middle cerebral vein
13. Middle cerebral artery
14. Anterior temporal artery (off posterior cerebral artery)
15. Deep temporal arterial branch (off maxillary artery), deep temporal nerve (off motor root of V3), and vein in temporalis muscle
16. Zygomatic arch
17. Greater and lesser palatine nerves descending within palatine canal(s) from pterygopalatine fossa to oral cavity
18. Parotid duct, buccal branch of facial nerve
19. Masseter muscle
20. Facial vein
21. Inferior alveolar nerve, artery, and vein inside mandibular canal
22. Left submandibular duct (superior) and lingual nerve (inferior) within sublingual gland
23. Submental artery and vein, submandibular gland
24. Geniohyoid muscles (right and left), septum of tongue
25. Digastric muscle
26. Mylohyoid muscle
27. Hypoglossal nerve (inferior), lingual artery (superior)
28. Right submandibular duct (superior) and lingual nerve (inferior) within sublingual gland
29. Facial artery
30. Inferior alveolar nerve, artery, and vein inside mandibular canal
31. Facial vein
32. Palatine glands in mucosa of hard palate, greater palatine nerve
33. Inferior alveolar artery, vein, and nerve headed toward mandibular foramen
34. Parotid duct, buccal branches of facial nerve, transverse facial artery
35. Coronoid process of mandible, masseter muscle
36. Inferior nasal concha (turbinate), nasal septum (vomer)
37. Temporalis muscle and maxillary artery in infratemporal fossa
38. Zygomatic arch and tendon of temporalis muscle
39. Maxillary nerve
40. Optic nerve and ophthalmic artery within optic canal
41. Superficial temporal artery and vein (frontal branches)
42. Anterior clinoid process
43. Temporal lobe of brain
44. Middle meningeal artery (frontal branch)
45. Gyrus rectus, olfactory tract
46. Inferior frontal gyrus of cerebral hemisphere
47. Anterior cerebral arteries
48. Middle frontal gyrus of cerebral hemisphere
49. Cingulate gyrus
50. Galea aponeurotica (extends from frontalis muscle)
51. Superior frontal gyrus
52. Arachnoid granulation
53. Lateral venous lacuna (outpouching of superior sagittal sinus)—note the pit in inner surface of the skull caused by arachnoid granulation
54. Body of tongue
55. Oral cavity
56. Nasal cavity (left)
57. Sphenoid sinuses (right and left), septum
58. Cranial nerves III, IV, VI, ophthalmic nerve, and superior ophthalmic vein in cavernous sinus
59. Pterygopalatine ganglion

1_____
2_____
3_____
4_____
5_____
6_____
7_____
8_____
9_____
10_____
11_____
12_____
13_____
14_____
15_____
16_____
17_____
18_____
19_____
20_____
21_____
22_____
23_____
24_____
25_____
26_____
27_____
28_____
29_____
30_____
31_____
32_____
33_____

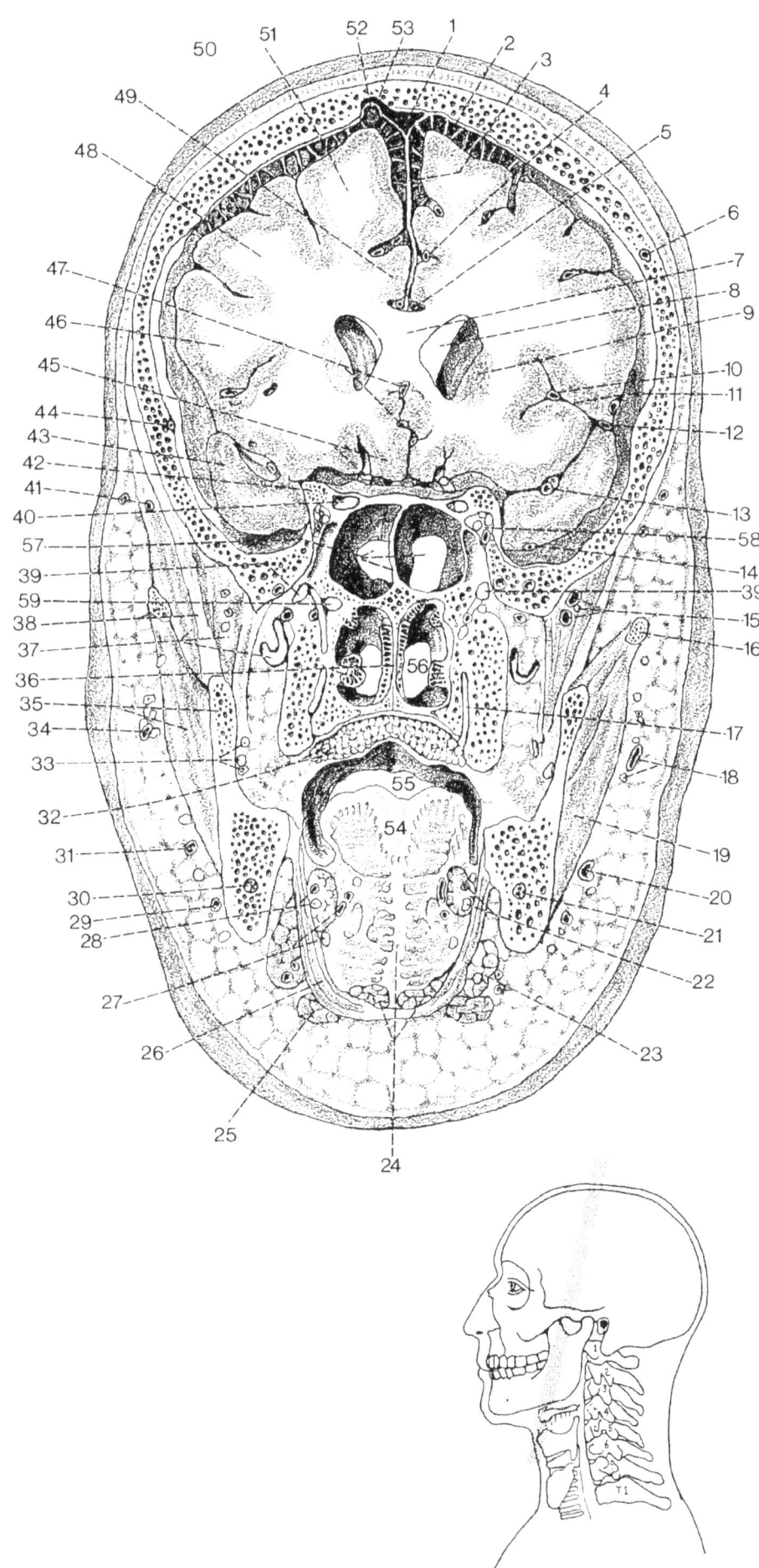

34 _____
35 _____
36 _____
37 _____
38 _____
39 _____
40 _____
41 _____
42 _____
43 _____
44 _____
45 _____
46 _____
47 _____
48 _____
49 _____
50 _____
51 _____
52 _____
53 _____
54 _____
55 _____
56 _____
57 _____
58 _____
59 _____

157

H&N-92 Optic chiasm level

Color and label

1. Sagittal suture (between parietal bones)
2. Falx cerebri
3. Pericallosal artery (continuation of anterior cerebral artery)
4. Corpus callosum
5. Septum pellucidum (the two septa appear to be fused together)
6. Lateral ventricle (left)
7. Squamosal suture (between temporal and parietal bones)
8. Lateral fissure (of Sylvius; in brain)
9. Middle cerebral artery
10. Internal carotid artery (cut at 10 and again at 12, here as part of circle of Willis)
11. Oculomotor nerve (in lateral wall of cavernous sinus)
12. Internal carotid artery (here coursing forward within cavernous sinus)
13. Abducens nerve (above) and maxillary nerve (below)
14. Middle meningeal artery and vein (doubled)
15. Zygomatic process of temporal bone
16. Lateral pterygoid muscle, nerve to lateral pterygoid (from the motor portion of the trigeminal nerve), branches of maxillary artery
17. Masseter muscle
18. Buccal nerve (sensory branch of mandibular nerve)
19. Parotid duct (over or above buccal branch of mandibular nerve)
20. Inferior alveolar nerve and artery in mandibular canal
21. Medial pterygoid muscle
22. Nerve to mylohyoid muscle
23. Lingual nerve (lateral), styloglossus muscle (medial)
24. Facial vein with mandibular branch of facial nerve
25. Facial artery
26. Submandibular duct
27. Submandibular gland
28. Hypoglossal nerve (lateral) and lingual artery (medial), separated by hyoglossus muscle
29. Infrahyoid muscles (strap muscles of the neck)
30. Cricothyroid muscle
31. Thyroid cartilage
32. Sublingual glands (right and left)
33. Hyoid bone
34. Mylohyoid muscle
35. Lingual artery (medial), submandibular gland (lateral)
36. Hyoglossus muscle
37. Lingual septum, intrinsic tongue muscles
38. Lingual nerve (lateral), styloglossus muscle (medial)
39. Uvula (in midline) and underside of soft palate
40. Mylohyoid nerve (also supplies anterior belly of diagastric muscle)
41. Inferior alveolar artery, vein, and nerve in mandibular canal
42. Tensor veli palatini muscle, lesser palatine nerve and vessels
43. Levator veli palatini muscle
44. Parotid duct, buccal branch of facial nerve
45. Posterior wall of nasopharynx (site of pharyngeal tonsil) viewed through posterior aperature of nasal cavity (choanae)
46. Auditory (eustachian) tube—cartilaginous part
47. Zygomatic arch (zygomatic process of temporal bone)
48. Sphenoidal sinus and septum
49. Pituitary gland (hypophysis) in sella turcica, infundibulum (pituitary stalk)
50. Optic chiasm
51. Squamosal suture
52. Anterioir cerebral arteries
53. Superior sagittal sinus
54. Soft palate (sectioned)
55. Middle cerebral artery (above), anterior clinoid process (below)
56. Middle cerebral artery
57. Medial pterygoid plate
58. Lateral pterygoid plate (note how thin they are)

1 _____
2 _____
3 _____
4 _____
5 _____
6 _____
7 _____
8 _____
9 _____
10 _____
11 _____
12 _____
13 _____
14 _____
15 _____
16 _____
17 _____
18 _____
19 _____
20 _____
21 _____
22 _____
23 _____
24 _____
25 _____
26 _____
27 _____
28 _____
29 _____
30 _____
31 _____
32 _____
33 _____

34 _____
35 _____
36 _____
37 _____
38 _____
39 _____
40 _____
41 _____
42 _____
43 _____
44 _____
45 _____
46 _____
47 _____
48 _____
49 _____
50 _____
51 _____
52 _____
53 _____
54 _____
55 _____
56 _____
57 _____
58 _____

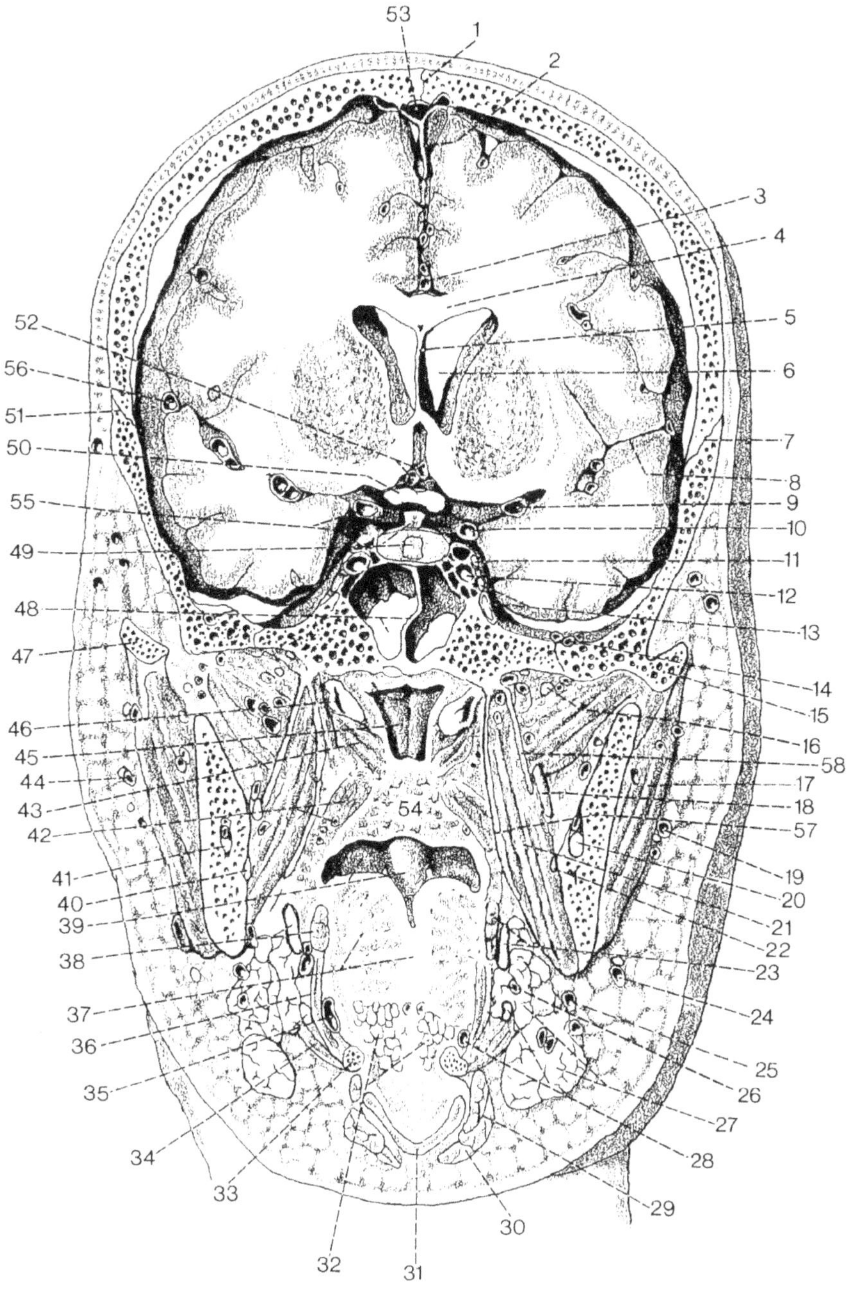

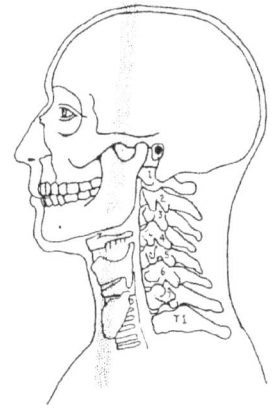

H&N-93 Carotid canal level

Color and label

1. Supeior sagittal sinus
2. Falx cerebri
3. Cingulate gyrus
4. Corpus callosum
5. Lateral ventricle
6. Septum pellucidum (right and left fused together)
7. Fornix (body)—both right and left
8. Ventricle III
9. Superficial temporal artery
10. Inferior (temporal) horn of lateral ventricle
11. Trigeminal ganglion
12. Internal carotid artery in carotid canal in temporal bone
13. Superficial temporal artery
14. Auriculotemporal nerve (medial) and small part of mandible head (lateral)
15. Maxillary vein
16. Parotid duct
17. Parotid gland
18. Pharyngeal constrictor muscles
19. Hyoid bone
20. Posterior wall of pharynx
21. Arytenoid cartilage
22. Thyroid cartilage
23. Cricoid cartilage
24. Cricothyroid muscle
25. Sternocleidomastoid muscle (clavicular head)
26. Clavicle (left)
27. Sternothyroid and sternohyoid muscles
28. Infraglottic space (below the vocal folds)—back wall is mucosa-lined lamina of the cricoid cartilage
29. Thyroid gland (right lateral lobe)
30. Clavicle (right)
31. Thyroarytenoid muscle
32. Thyrohyoid muscle
33. Thyrohyoid membrane (white band between thyroid cartilage and hyoid bone)
34. Superior laryngeal nerve (branch of N X)
35. Submandibular gland
36. Hypoglossal nerve (N XII)
37. Intermediate tendon of digastric muscle (connects its two bellies)
38. Stylohyoid muscle
39. Stylopharyngeus muscle and glossopharyngeal nerve (N IX)
40. Styloglossus muscle
41. Anterior tubercle of atlas (C1), longus capitis muscle
42. Parotid duct within parotid gland
43. Body of sphenoid bone (posterior part)
44. Auriculotemporal nerve and maxillary artery
45. Head of mandible (right side)
46. Superficial temporal artery
47. Articular disk inside temporomandibular joint
48. Internal carotid artery (right) in carotid canal
49. Basilar artery on ventral surface of pons of brain stem
50. Oculomotor nerve (N III)
51. Lateral (Sylvian) cerebral fissure with middle cerrebral artery
52. Sternohyoid muscle
53. Branches of facial nerve in parotid gland
54. Sternothyroid muscle
55. First tracheal ring
56. Maxillary artery

1_____
2_____
3_____
4_____
5_____
6_____
7_____
8_____
9_____
10_____
11_____
12_____
13_____
14_____
15_____
16_____
17_____
18_____
19_____
20_____
21_____
22_____
23_____
24_____
25_____
26_____
27_____
28_____
29_____
30_____
31_____
32_____
33_____
34_____
35_____
36_____

37 _____
38 _____
39 _____
40 _____
41 _____
42 _____
43 _____
44 _____
45 _____
46 _____
47 _____
48 _____
49 _____
50 _____
51 _____
52 _____
53 _____
54 _____
55 _____
56 _____

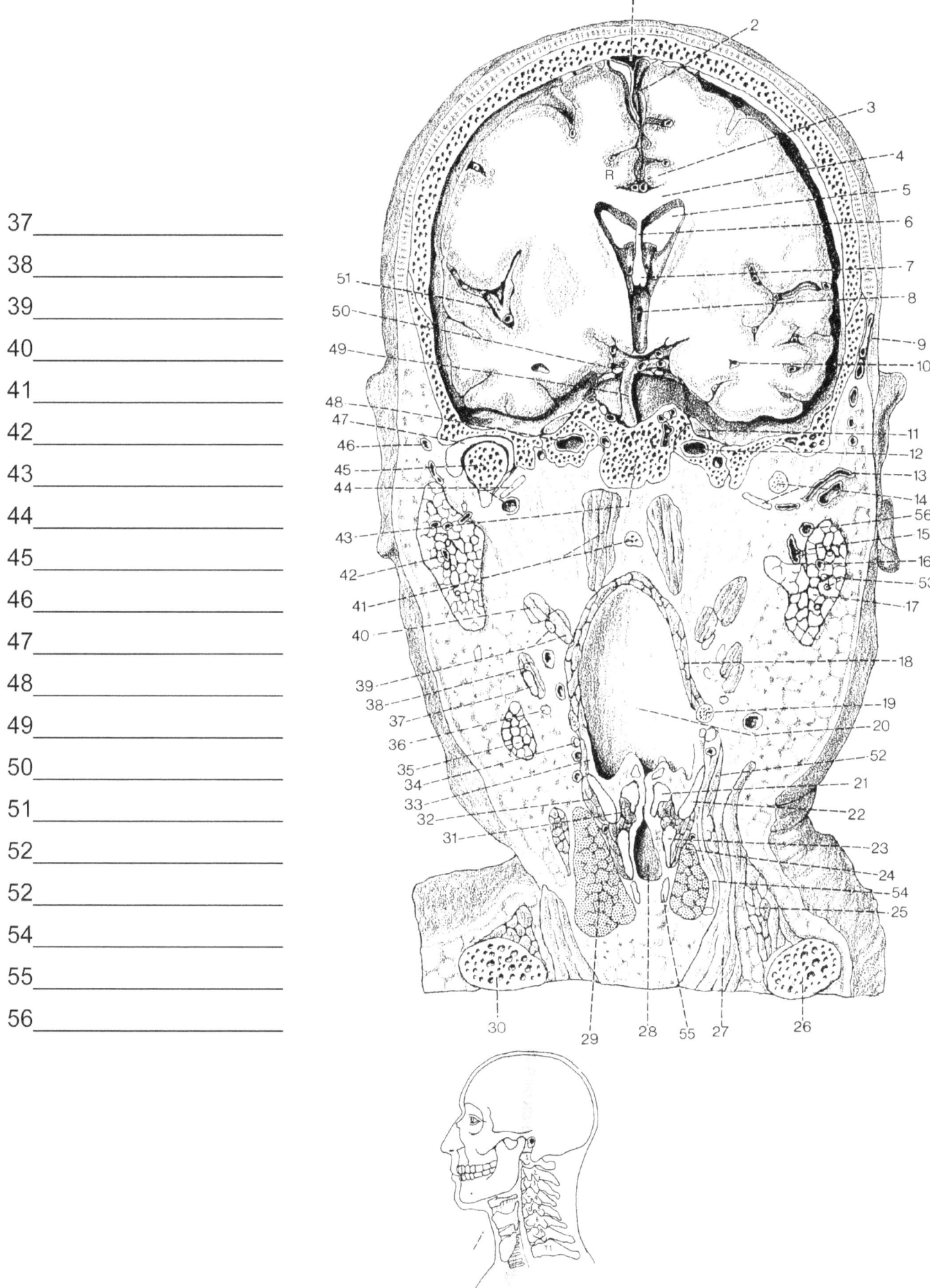

H&N-94 Pons, internal jugular vein level

Color and label

1. Superior sagittal sinus
2. Falx cerebri
3. Cingulate gyrus
4. Corpus callosum
5. Left lateral ventricle
6. Fornix
7. Lateral (Sylvian) fissure
8. Superior temporal gyrus
9. Inferior (temporal) horn of left lateral ventricle
10. Middle temporal gyrus
11. Inferior temporal gyrus
12. Edge of tentorium cerebelli
13. Facial nerve and vestibulocochlear nerve in internal auditory (acoustic) meatus
14. Air cells in temporal bone
15. Vestibule (cavity containing utricle and saccule) of inner ear
16. External auditory meatus (ear canal)
17. Left hypoglossal nerve (N XII) in hypoglossal canal
18. Facial nerve (N VII) descending through facial canal in petrous temporal bone
19. Occipital condyle
20. Facial nerve branches within parotid gland
21. Parotid duct within parotid gland
22. Atlanto-occipital joint (joint between vertebra C1 and occipital condyles at base of skull)
23. Odontoid process (dens) of C2 (axis)
24. Dorsal root ganglion of cervical spinal nerve C2
25. Internal jugular vein (left)—cut in several places
26. Internal carotid artery
27. Maxillary vein
28. Sternocleidomastoid muscle
29. Common carotid artery (left)
30. Thoracic duct
31. Clavicle (left)
32. Subclavian vein
33. Esophagus
34. Lymph glands
35. Thyroid gland
36. Clavicle (right)
37. Internal jugular vein (right)
38. Common carotid artery (right)
39. Sympathetic trunk (right)
40. Vagus nerve (right)
41. Longus colli muscle
42. Cervical vertebra C3
43. Cervical vertebra C2
44. Atlanto-axial joint (joint between cervical vertebrae C1 and C2) and right vagus nerve (N X)
45. Stylohyoid ligament and stylohyoid muscle
46. Internal jugular vein (right)
47. Parotid duct and facial nerve branches in parotid gland
48. Basilar artery on ventral medulla
49. Hypoglossal nerve (right)
50. Facial nerve (right) within facial canal
51. Tympanic cavity (middle ear, lateral) and cochlea (medial)
52. Nerves VII (facial) and VIII (vestibulocochlear, right) entering internal auditory meatus
53. Vestibule of right inner ear
54. Epitympanic recess (upper compartment of middle ear)
55. Pons
56. Middle meningeal artery
57. Hippocampal formation within temporal lobe of brain
58. Substantia nigra of midbrain
59. Ventricle III
60. Jugular foramen

1 _____
2 _____
3 _____
4 _____
5 _____
6 _____
7 _____
8 _____
9 _____
10 _____
11 _____
12 _____
13 _____
14 _____
15 _____
16 _____
17 _____
18 _____
19 _____
20 _____
21 _____
22 _____
23 _____
24 _____
25 _____
26 _____
27 _____
28 _____
29 _____
30 _____
31 _____
32 _____
33 _____

34 ___
35 ___
36 ___
37 ___
38 ___
39 ___
40 ___
41 ___
42 ___
43 ___
44 ___
45 ___
46 ___
47 ___
48 ___
49 ___
50 ___
51 ___
52 ___
53 ___
54 ___
55 ___
56 ___
57 ___
58 ___
59 ___
60 ___

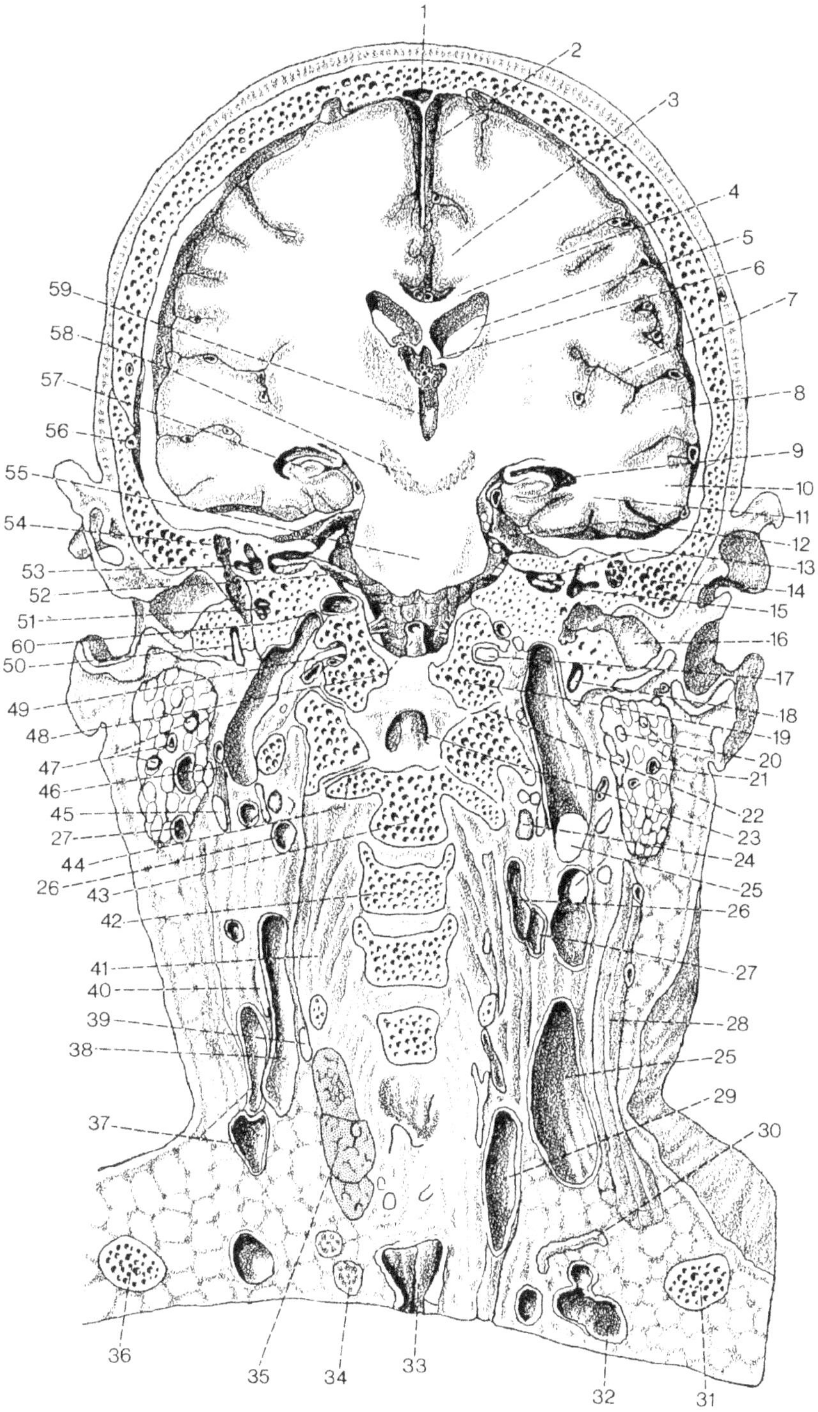

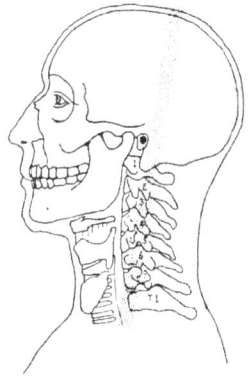

H&N-95 Dens of axis level

Color and label

1. Superior sagittal sinus
2. Lateral lacuna (outpouching) of superior sagittal sinus
3. Falx cerebri
4. Diploic vein
5. Cingulate gyrus
6. Pericallosal arteries (continuation of anterior cerebral arteries)
7. Corpus callosum
8. Lateral ventricle
9. Fornix
10. Pineal gland
11. Inferior (temporal) horn of lateral ventricle and choroid plexus
12. Ventricle IV (narrow superior end approaching cerebral aqueduct)
13. Tentorium cerebelli
14. Superior petrosal sinus
15. Cerebellar hemisphere
16. Sigmoid sinus
17. Lesser occipital nerve
18. Mastoid air cells in mastoid process
19. Odontoid process (dens) of cervical vertebra C2
20. Accessory nerve (N XI)
21. Vertebral artery (left)
22. Great auricular nerve (cutaneous branch of cervical plexus)
23. External jugular vein
24. Spinal ganglion (dorsal root ganglion) of spinal nerve; C3 in intervetebral foramen
25. Spinal cord (anterior surface); note anterior rootlets of spinal nerves
26. Portion of posterior wall of internal jugular vein
27. Sternocleidomastoid muscle
28. Vertebra C5 body
29. Spinal nerve C6
30. Vertebral artery
31. Scalenus medius muscle
32. Clavicle (left)
33. Subclavian artery
34. First rib
35. Vertebra C6 body
36. Esophagus
37. Vertebra C7 body
38. Vertebral artery (right)
39. Brachial plexus
40. Clavicle (right)
41. Vertebra C5 transverse process
42. Ventral rootlets (right) coalescing into ventral root of spinal nerve C5
43. Vertebra C4 transverse process
44. Denticulate (toothlike) ligament
45. Anterior spinal artery
46. Accessory nerve N XI (right)
47. Vertebra C3 transverse process
48. Vertebra C2 transverse process and right vertebral artery
49. Spinal nerve C2 with its dural sheath
50. Atlanto-occipital joint (between skull and C1 vertebra), transverse process of C1 (atlas)
51. Occipital condyle
52. Middle cerebellar peduncle (formerly brachium pontis Latin, arm of the pons)
53. Superior colliculus of midbrain
54. Internal cerebral veins (join posteriorly to form great cerebral vein of Galen)
55. Splenium of corpus callosum
56. Artifactual space caused by collapse of arachnoid membrane onto pia mater and obliteration of subarachnoid space—normally arachnoid membrane rests directly inside dura mater. A subdural hematoma would form in this potential space.
57. Arachnoid granulation (stretched and distorted)
58. Medulla oblongata
59. Anterior scalene muscle

1_____
2_____
3_____
4_____
5_____
6_____
7_____
8_____
9_____
10_____
11_____
12_____
13_____
14_____
15_____
16_____
17_____
18_____
19_____
20_____
21_____
22_____
23_____
24_____
25_____
26_____
27_____
28_____
29_____
30_____
31_____
32_____
33_____
34_____
35_____
36_____

(use abbrevs.)

37 _____
38 _____
39 _____
40 _____
41 _____
42 _____
43 _____
44 _____
45 _____
46 _____
47 _____
48 _____
49 _____
50 _____
51 _____
52 _____
53 _____
54 _____
55 _____
56 _____
57 _____
58 _____
59 _____

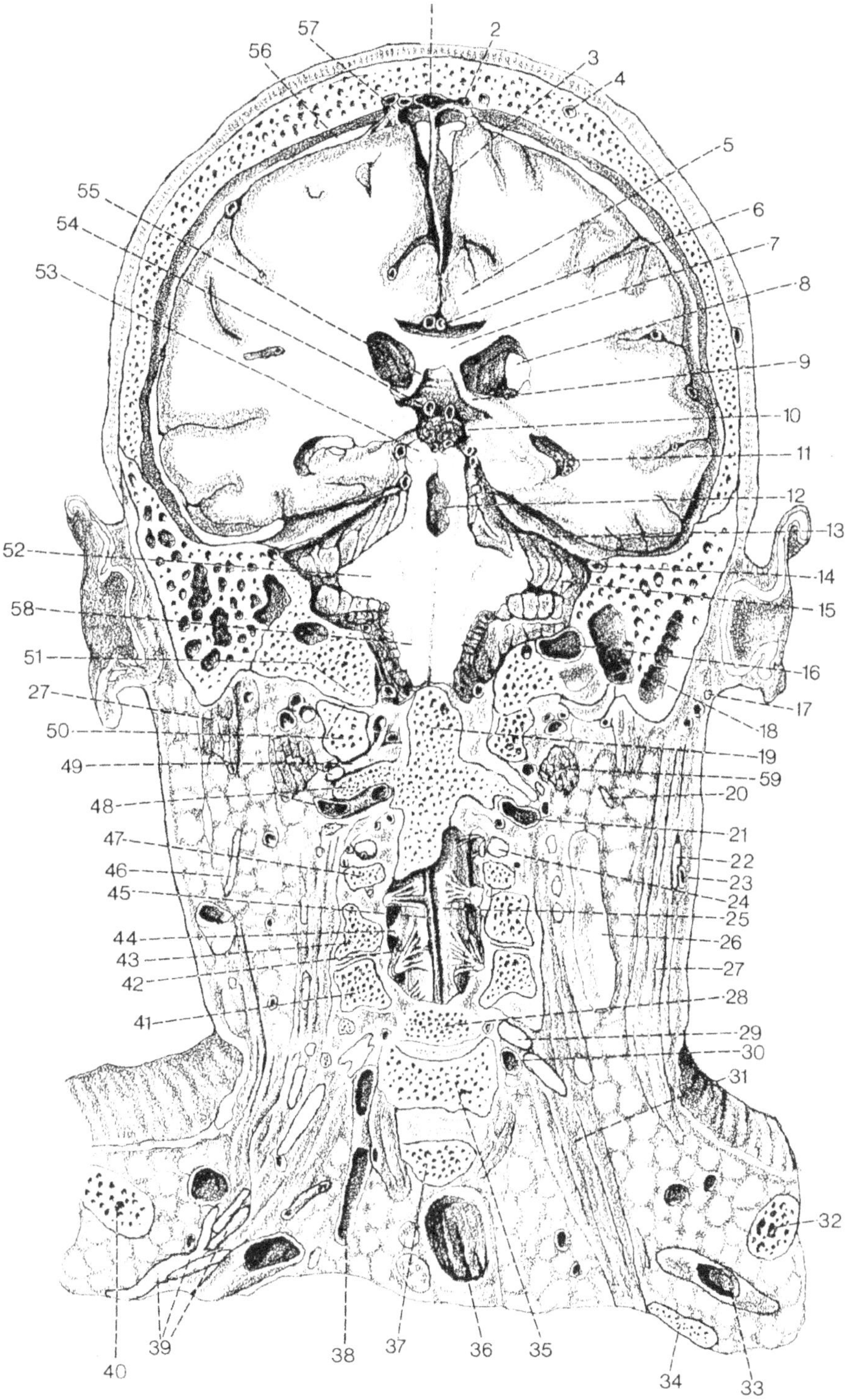

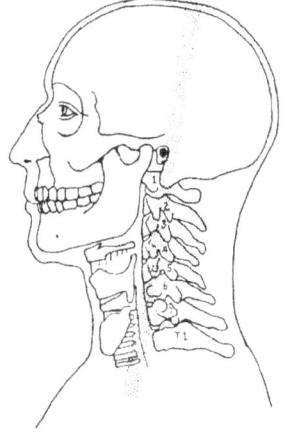

165

H&N-1 Head and Neck

Trigemini
(Triplets)

Trigemini is Latin for "triplets." The trigeminal nerve is named the triplet nerve because it divides into three large nerves, the ophthalmic nerve, the maxillary nerve, and the mandibular nerve.

Gemini means "twins" and *quadrigemini* is "quadruplets."

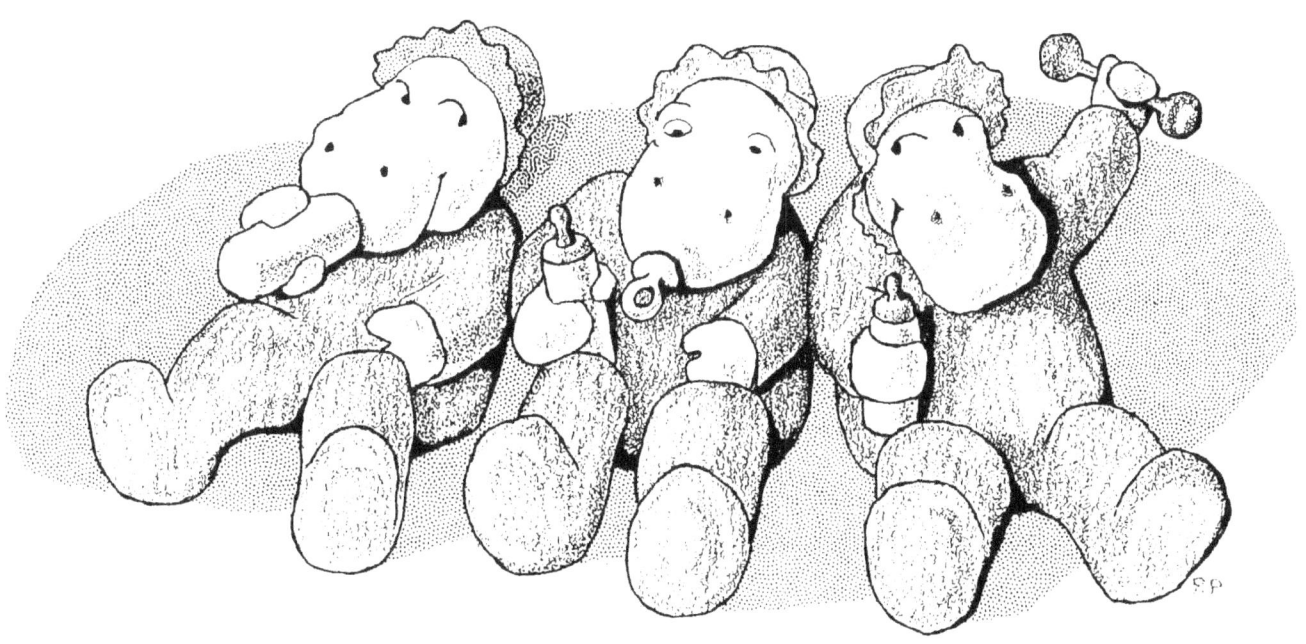

www.ingramcontent.com/pod-product-compliance
Lightning Source LLC
Chambersburg PA
CBHW081217230426

43666CB00015B/2763